Tai Ji Foundations
武式太極拳

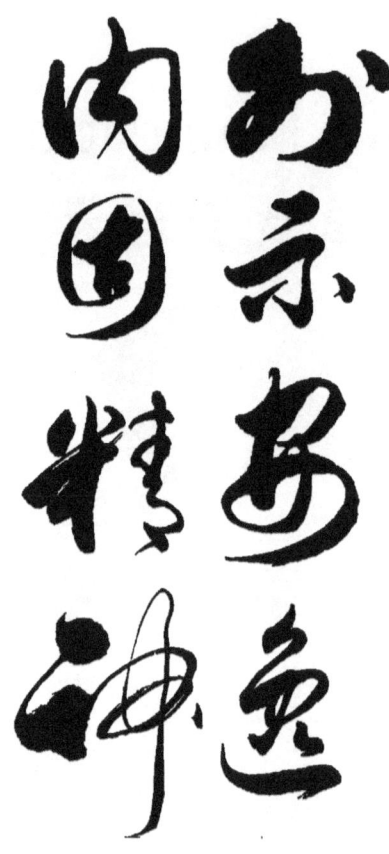

EXTERNALLY AT EASE

———————

INTERNALIZE THE SPIRIT

Tai Ji Foundations
武式太極拳

TRANSLATION AND COMMENTARY
PANG CHAOSUN

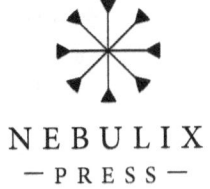

NEBULIX
—PRESS—

ISBN 979-8-9897252-9-8 (SOFT COVER)
ISBN 979-8-9897252-7-4 (HARD COVER)
ISBN 979-8-9897252-8-1 (E-BOOK)

Second Edition
Printed in the United States

scan for speaking engagements,
seminars, bulk purchase,
and other inquiries

www.sbwuhaotaiji.com

CREDITS
Gabriella Klein, Editorial Support
Zheng YingPing, Calligraphy · **Kevin Gleason,** Ilustrations
Jane Gottlieb, Photo Touch Up · **Noah Pang,** Technical Assistance
John Balkwill / Lumino Press, Book Design

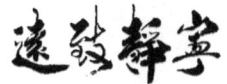

To Go Far, First Be Still

Chinese Proverb
139 BC

Table of Contents

CHAPTER THREE
INNER WORKINGS OF WU STYLE
TAI JI QUAN PRACTICE

CHAPTER FOUR
WU STYLE TAI JI QUAN FORMS

CHAPTER FIVE
WU STYLE TAI JI QUAN STRIKING HANDS PRACTICE

CHAPTER SIX

Manuscripts by Wang ZongYue, Wu YuXiang, and Li YiYu

---

1. There is some uncertainty as to who wrote the Thirteen Principles Practice Sonnet, Wang ZongYue or Wu YuXiang

Epilogue

Acknowledgements

There are several people whom I would like to thank, for without their dedication and commitment, this book would not have come to fruition. First among them is my wife Gin for being so understanding and willing to study Tai Ji together with me for all these years, and for providing insights when I was unable to understand. I would also like to thank Julia Emerson for her tireless work, patience and perseverance while editing my manuscript and for her encouragement in helping me to complete this book. Many thanks also to Jane Gottlieb for the photographic touch-ups, to Noah Pang for his assistance with the figures, to Mr. Zheng YinPing for his calligraphy, to Kevin Gleason for his illustrations and to Gabriella Klein for her careful reading of the manuscript. Thanks also to John Balkwill and Chryss Yost for tackling this project with such skill and curiosity. Finally, my thanks to Susan Tai for her generous support over the years.

武式郝家太极拳師承表
Wu Style Hao Family Tai Ji Lineage

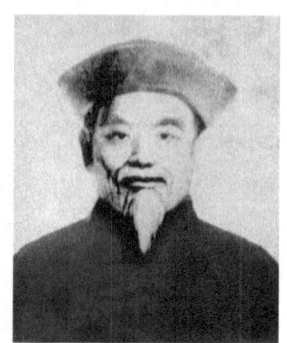

武禹襄 Wu YuXiang
1812-1880

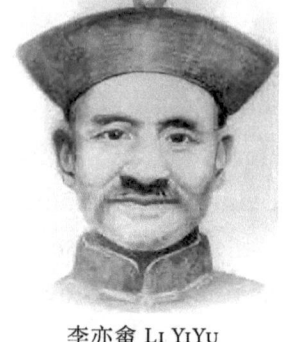

李亦畬 Li YiYu
1832-1892

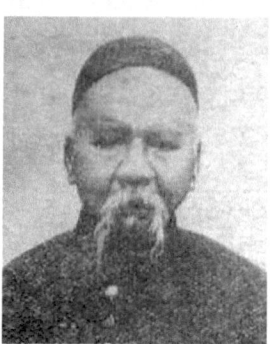

郝為真 Hao WeiZhen
1849-1920

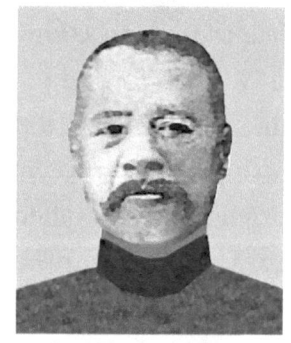

郝月如 Hao YueRu
1887-1935

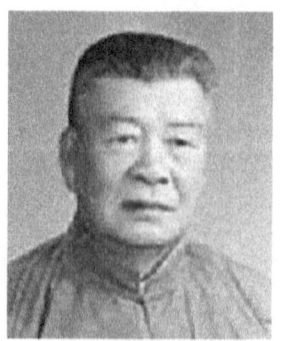

郝少如 Hao ShaoRu
1906-1983

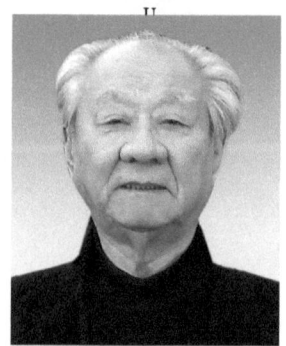

劉積順 Liu JiShun
1930-

INTRODUCTION
Pang ChaoSun

WITH THE WORLD SLOWING down during the pandemic of 2020, I had the extra time at home to improve my Tai Ji skills without outside distractions. The book *Wu Style Tai Ji Quan*, written by Hao ShaoRu, was a constant companion, allowing me to gain insight into this marvelous art. Before the pandemic I had already translated a portion of the book for my students so they could use the instructions for their own practice. With the extra time, I was able to finish translating the entire book into English.

There were other challenges that had kept me from pursuing the translation. First, it is difficult to translate some of the older forms of the Chinese language used in the writings because there is no equivalent in contemporary Chinese. It is even more difficult to find equivalent language in English. In addition, I questioned my ability to describe these abstract concepts clearly. This challenge was mostly resolved by teaching Tai Ji for close to two decades to both beginners and advanced students. Through trial and error, I was able to build a bridge with words between two very different ways of looking at the world, Eastern and Western. Surprisingly, the second challenge was resolved by translating this book. I had read *Wu Style Tai Ji Quan* many times and pondered the details. However, during translation there was a constant struggle over the best way to express what had been written. This struggle, combined with Master Liu's teaching and my personal practice, allowed the words to start to make sense to me and gave me confidence. Although this book is based on Hao ShaoRu's book *Wu Style Tai Ji Quan*, to make it more readable and comprehensible in English, I have taken the liberty of reorganizing and restructuring the book. Nevertheless, there still are poetic passages that I left as close to the original as possible, particularly in Chapter 6, which contains the translation of the original handwritten copy of the *Tai Ji Manual* by Li YiYu. Hao ShaoRu mentions many times in his book that Tai Ji Quan is an art, and that, as with any art, it sometimes is best to leave the reader room to imagine and be creative in finding a path of their own for this practice.

PURPOSE

Wu Style Tai Ji Quan is currently also called Wu Style Hao Family Tai Ji Quan (Wu Hao). It is recognized as one of the five unique Tai Ji Quan styles practiced today. The others are Chen, Yang, Wu[1] and Sun Style Tai Ji Quan[2]. The major contribution of Wu Hao Style Tai Ji Quan is the valuable written source material that provides the theoretical foundations which include the *Tai Ji Classic* and the treatise written by Wang ZongYue, and as well as commentary and

1 Chinese is a tonal language with five tones, there is often confusion among people who do not speak Chinese about how to enunciate Wu (武). To further the confusion, there is a Wu (吳) Style Tai Ji which is a derivation of Yang Style and which was created by a student of Yang Lu Chan. 武 is a lower, or third tone in Wu Hao Tai Ji, while 吳 is a higher, second tone.
2 I have a more detailed description of the Wu Hao history in the Epilogue.

insights by Wu, Li, and three generations of Hao masters. These are among the earliest original source materials and are used extensively by practitioners of all Tai Ji styles, and by other internal martial arts for reference and for pondering. The purpose of this book is to provide a reference source in English for Tai Ji Quan practitioners who want to have a deeper understanding of the terminology and internal techniques but who are not familiar with the Chinese language.

Wu Style Tai Ji Quan, written in Chinese by Hao ShaoRu, presents many of the Tai Ji concepts such as Open and Converge, Let Go of Oneself and Follow Others, and insights such as how the energy initiates at the foot, is expressed in the legs, is controlled by the waist and forms at the fingers. Body Principles such as Relax the Chest, Open the Back, and Suspend the Head all originated with writings by Wu YuXiang and were further expanded upon by Li YiYu with his five Key Words: Heart Calm, Body Intuitive (Agile), Qi Converged, Jin Unified and Spirit Gathered. In addition, three generations of Hao family members added explanations such as: Spacious, Relaxed, Round and Lively, Methods of Folding, Five Bows, Tai Ji Breathing and others. As the concepts became more commonplace, very few knew the original source of the teachings. Sometimes the teachings were wrongly attributed to other authors, and they were often quoted without knowing the full context. Differences in language and culture have led to the information being further diluted and misunderstood when it is taught in the West. Conveying the wisdom of the ancient *Tai Ji Classic* to the modern practitioner is a complex subject even for Chinese speakers. It is even more difficult in another language. In addition, many of the teachers, when they began teaching foreigners, used the most simplistic vocabulary and expressions for the sake of expediency. Thus, they were unable to convey the nuances of the theories of Tai Ji Quan. There is also the problem of translations by people who do not practice the Wu Hao Style. They lack knowledge of the inner workings and might lead readers down an erroneous path.

I have studied many martial arts of both the East and the West as well as three different styles of Tai Ji over many years. However, it is when I studied Wu Hao family style in depth over a couple of decades that I finally was able to come to a fuller understanding of what is possible. As each skill is acquired, each word in the *Tai Ji Classic* starts to come to life and take on meaning. It is this that motivates me to write this book and share the knowledge. Although my English is far from perfect, I have lived in the United States since I was thirteen, and I have taught the subject matter for over two decades. This, combined with the editing skills of my senior student Julia Emerson, puts me in a good position to convey the information in these foundational texts to the reader in English. It has been a painstaking process. For instance, Wu Hao Style is known in China to emphasize the energy of opening and converging. However, it is often called Open and Close Style in English. The Chinese character 開, is translated as open in English and consequently the other word, 合, has been translated as close, because close is the opposite of open. However, I have chosen to use the word converge instead of close, because "open" in Wu Hao Tai Ji implies the sensation of openness combined with expansion, and therefore "converge" is a better word to convey the opposing force. It is this level of attention to detail that has guided me in this translation.

I have decided to use Tai Ji rather than Tai Chi, and instead of Chi, I use Qi for this book. This is not to confuse the reader but rather to show that the modern Pinyin system clarifies a difference between Ji (極) and Qi (氣) that is readily apparent in Chinese. Tai Ji (太極) is composed of Tai, meaning beyond, and Ji, meaning limits. Together they reference the Chinese understanding of the cosmos as a duality of Yin and Yang with limitless manifestations rather than as a linear system with limits. Qi literally means air in Chinese, indicating an energetic, flowing sensation in the body.

Here, I want to thank the founders of Wu Hao Tai Ji Quan for not having kept their methods and insights a secret. There are three reasons why this information became widely available in Chinese. First, Wu and Li both were scholars who had the ability to describe their practice with precision, using the appropriate words. Second, they were wealthy and did not depend on teaching Tai Ji Quan to make a living. For them it was a lifetime hobby as well as a way of maintaining their physical health. They did treat this as precious information but were willing to share with others who wanted to learn. That is why this information was passed on to the Hao Family. The information was also shared with the Yang family, especially through one of Yang LuChan's sons, Yang BanHou who studied with Wu directly. Third, Hao ShaoRu was able to organize all the original texts, along with the original manuscripts from Wu and Li, into the book *Wu Style Tai Ji Quan*. This book contains detailed explanations as well as the knowledge and insight that the Hao family gained through three generations.

In this book, I also want to leave room for the reader to imagine even greater possibilities, so that others may achieve heights beyond my understanding. Therefore, in Chapter 6, for some of the most ancient writings by Wang ZongYue, I have provided the original Chinese text along with my best effort at translation and without commentary. Consequently, future generations may be able to translate the original Chinese text with even greater clarity.

UNDERSTANDING WU HAO TAI JI QUAN

Tai Ji Quan is a martial art as well as a healing art and is based on the Chinese philosophical understanding of the theory of Yin Yang. There is a considerable amount of specialized terminology that is difficult to translate because it defies simple, direct explanations. As Lao Zi said in the *Dao De Jing*: "From One comes Two and from Two comes Three and from Three come all things." Therefore, in Chinese culture, all phenomena (the One) have at least two different aspects, Yin and Yang, and the third is a combination of the two that created it. As you are reading the book, you must keep this in mind. Words such as Qi have a multitude of meanings depending on the context in which they are used. In China, this concept of duality drives every aspect of the culture, from art, literature and farming to relationships and medicine. It even extends to the functioning of government and conducting warfare. Tai Ji Quan is no exception. It is an example of how this philosophy manifests in our mind and body.

Wang ZongYue's *Tai Ji Treatise*[3] starts by mentioning that Tai Ji came from Wu Ji and is the mother of all things. Wu Ji

---

3 *Tai Ji Treatise*, located in Chapter 6.

is our natural state and Tai Ji is a way of describing this state using two complementary forces, Yin and Yang, the mother that makes all things possible. The Chinese also believe that there are three aspects to our being: Jing (精), the physical; Qi (氣), the emotions and feelings; and Shen (神), the mind and consciousness. All three need to work together to create a healthy life. This is described at the end of *Thirteen Principles Practice Sonnet*[4], which states that the goal of Tai Ji Quan is to assist the practitioner in living a good long life.

Let us consider the Yin Yang aspect of Jing, Qi and Shen that, as the mother, make up our being and allow us to function in the world. First, Jing is our physical being. The Yang aspect is the physical body composed of bone, muscles, sinews and organs. The Yin aspect is rest and the nutrients that nurture our body to keep it functioning. Therefore, using Lao Zi's metaphor, One is the body and Two is doing work (Yang) and resting and eating (Yin), and Three is working and resting and eating integrated in appropriate amounts to make a healthy being. To provide another analogy, if we look more closely at how the body moves, we can see that movement requires two different muscle groups: the extensors (Yang) and the contractors (Yin). Therefore, using Lao Zi's metaphor for movements, One is the physical body, Two is the contractor and extensor muscles, and Three is the appropriate amount of muscle contraction and extension to make movement possible.

To further illustrate the necessity of a balance between Yin and Yang energies, there is an ancient saying: "Too Yang is exhausting and too Yin is stagnant." The reason is that if you are too Yang and are working too much without rest and

---

4 *Thirteen Principles Practice Sonnet*, located in Chapter 6.

proper nutrients, the body will exhaust itself and cannot continue. The other way around, if you just eat and rest all the time, nothing ever gets done and you are stagnant.

Second, Qi is complicated and difficult to describe to the beginner. Even with many years of practice I still find a description of Qi elusive. When I first started to study Tai Ji, I thought Qi was a special energy that we develop and cultivate through Tai Ji practice and that, along with self-defense, this Qi energy could be used in interesting ways to keep our life force strong. I have a Tai Ji friend who is a biophysicist. Upon his retirement, he decided to use his laboratory of instruments to try to find Qi. After years of searching, he finally gave up and said to me that there are biomarkers such as the hands and body getting warmer and a general sense of well-being, but there is no unique substance in the electromagnetic spectrum or the physical manifestation that can be measured and is different from ordinary bodily functions. With this discovery, what my teacher had taught me finally sank in. Master Liu always says that Qi is a feeling that you create and follow. When you are at ease, of course your body feels warmer and all the movement seems to be in the flow. When you are in stress, your body tenses up and circulation decreases. This makes you feel colder, as if you are fighting your own body to move. Qi is simply how you feel rather than some magical power.

Coming from another direction, Qi in Chinese literally means air. Air appears in Western culture as one of the four elements, fire, water, earth and air, that, according to the ancient Greeks, make up the physical world. Air is different from the other three elements in that it is the only element that cannot be seen and can only be known by feeling, as when the wind blows on the body. However, as human beings we have many more sensations than just the feeling of the wind. Like all emotions, Qi will lead to a visceral sensation in the body. Therefore air, the feeling element in the West, functions similarly to Qi in the East.

In Tai Ji Quan practice we pursue the spacious and relaxed Yin aspect of Qi as well as the round and lively Yang aspect of Qi (flowing sensation)[5]. The flowing sensation can further include an outward, expanding flow or an inward, converging flow. The sensation of flow is similar to what one experiences when one is in water. As you swim, you have a sensation of water flowing around your body. When Yin and Yang flow appropriately, the body will create a spring-like Jin (勁- internal power) for physical motion. The spring-like sensation is "Movement in Stillness" (preparing to move) which is described in Chapter Two as one of the Thirteen Body Principles.

The last of the three is Shen, which is typically translated as Spirit. Spirit is defined in the dictionary as the non-physical aspect of our being, and it is difficult to understand. After many years of working with it, I finally realized that in Tai Ji Quan, Spirit represents our mental capabilities. The Yang quality of Shen is intention and the Yin quality is our consciousness or self-awareness. Without intention we cannot manifest and without self-awareness we cannot make corrections to our actions.

---

5 Spacious, relaxed, round and lively are described in Chapter 3.

In one of Wu YuXiang's writings about Tai Ji Quan[6], Shen (intention) is compared to a general, and Qi (feeling) is like a flag. The flag is a metaphor for communication during ancient warfare. To move the troops, the general would tell the flag-waver to point in a certain direction so the soldiers would know where to go. In Tai Ji Quan, Shen (intention) gives the order and Qi directs the body. What are those feelings? They are the feelings of being spacious, relaxed, round and lively. Tai Ji Quan training moves slowly during practice so that there is time for adjustments to be made and the qualities of spacious, relaxed, round and lively can be felt. After mastering this step, one can generate those sensations more efficiently and move at a natural pace.

Each chapter provides many hints for learning those sensations. The most fundamental are the descriptions in the Body Principles such as Relax the Chest, Relax the Shoulder, and Suspend the Head. Explanations of the principles, such as the position of the body, are related to the Yang aspect. What most people overlook is the feeling, or Yin, aspect. An example of the Yin aspect is found in the description for Relax the Chest: "The chest is above the heart. Do not push it outward. The chest must relax so that the Qi can go downward. Both shoulders should round slightly forward and converge, so that heart intention can deploy Qi." It contains both the physical Yang description of the chest not pushing outward and the shoulders rounding forward, followed by the Yin description of a relaxed chest with Qi flowing downward and the shoulders feeling rounder and connected to allow the Qi to move.

---

6 First and Second Explanations to the Thirteen Principles Sonnet found in Chapter 6.

In the book there are many metaphors such as "Qi Collected at the Waist." What does this mean? One of the explanations in Chapter 4 under the Example of Sequence with Body Principles describes it as, "Qi Collected at the Waist means opening and relaxing both shoulders with the intention of sinking the Qi down the back. Both shoulders can gather toward the vertebrae, letting Qi converge at the waist. When the Qi can be collected to the waist, it can fill the waist. When Qi fills the waist, the waist can take command." This describes a process of releasing tension from the back by opening and rounding the shoulders forward. Once the shoulder is opened, there is a gentle Qi-like opposite sensation pulling toward the vertebrae rather than physically moving the shoulder toward the vertebrae. At this point, visualize a water-like feeling flowing down the back to the waist, creating an energy space around the waist near the physical center of the body. This Qi sensation creates an energetic feeling around the core of the body, where all movement must initiate, and is thus able to take command.

In this book, you will often encounter words such as gathering, converging, condensing, and closing which describe a kinesthetic sensation of Qi flowing inward, while words such as expressing, opening, radiating, and expanding describe a kinesthetic sensation of Qi flowing outward. In addition, other words such as nurturing the Qi refer to where the inward and outward Qi flows intermingle and generate a supporting, suspended sensation for the body as it prepares to move.

Another idiom, "Move Qi through the pearl with nine holes," also seems mysterious. It comes from a story about Confucius when he was trying to travel to another country.

The king did not want him to leave and challenged him to solve a puzzle to win permission to leave. The king gave him a pearl with nine holes and asked him to pull a thread through all nine holes. Confucius was unable to solve the puzzle until he met a woman who worked as a silkworm farmer. She showed him a way to solve the puzzle by tying a silk thread to an ant and, using honey as bait, leading the ant through the different holes to finish the puzzle. This metaphor implies that during practice you need to have the sensation of Qi throughout every pore in your body while still feeling connected like the thread through the pearl.

The terms substantial and insubstantial are also intriguing. Substantial is the word usually used to describe the foot one uses to generate power from the ground. This is a very limited view of substantiality. A broader view sees the body as substantial (Yang) and the energy space that we occupy by generating Qi flow as insubstantial (Yin). It is the Yin having the reserve potential for work that allows the Yang to perform work. In Tai Ji Quan it is the Qi flow that supports the body and allows it to move effortlessly, as a unit, in space.

How can insubstantial Qi support your body? The best example is a sprinter on the starting line. His body is still. His intention is on the distance ahead of him. There is a feeling (Qi) that something in front of him is drawing his body forward even before motion begins. The body at this point will feel light and ready to move. This is different from just holding a posture without any intention of moving. That body will feel heavier and unable to move spontaneously. With the sound of the bell, the sprinter's body will move to the intended place ahead of him purely through feeling, and each subsequent step will also be led by this energy to accelerate. Therefore, it is the insubstantial energy (forward intention combined with Qi sensation) that leads the substantial (body movement). What is interesting is that during this motion the body is light and Qi like, what athletes describe as "being in the flow," for efficient movement. In Wu Hao Tai Ji we call this, "preparing to move." Before movement commences there is movement in stillness, and the ability to use it in motion is called expressing Jin.

The difference between a sprinter and a Tai Ji practitioner is that the sprinter only creates a leading energy space in front of him, whereas the Tai Ji practitioner creates a uniform energy body all around himself so he can react and move in any direction in an instant. If one can move in any direction with equal energy, this implies there must be a center from which the energy can be equally distributed. It seems logical to assume that the center of our body (lower belly) should be this energy center. However, based on the structure of our body, the physical body should be behind the energy center for physical motion to have maximum power, as in the case of the sprinter. This system that includes mental intention, Qi sensation of the energy space, and the physical body is what Lao Zi called the One, and it contains the Two: Yin (energy space) and Yang (body) with the Three: the exchanges and transformation of the two to generate internal power (Jin).

Chapter 4, which describes the sequence of the 96 Forms for Wu Hao Tai Ji practice, needs to be carefully read. In addition to describing how to make each move physically, Hao ShaoRu has taken the additional step of providing notes and instructions describing how, in each form, intention and Qi should flow.

Readers should also note that the duality of Yin and Yang is relative. Yin can become Yang and Yang can become Yin, depending on the situation. Many practitioners are stuck in their practice because they understand Yin and Yang as absolutes rather than their being interchangeable and able to transform. In Chapter One under Transformation of Yin and Yang, Hao ShaoRu has written specifically to remind practitioners of this duality of meaning.

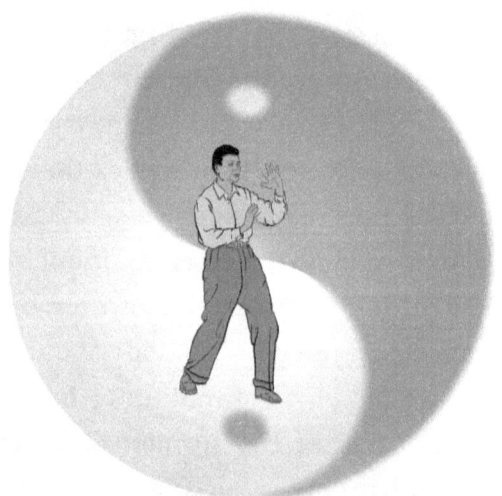

Finally, some of you might notice that the Yin Yang symbol is reverse in the diagram above, with white on the bottom and black on top. This is the result of an insight I had related to the practice of Tai Ji and the message of the Yi Jing (Book of Changes). According to the Yi Jing, there is a pre-heaven configuration that depicts the working of the cosmos and a post-heaven configuration showing how it manifests in humanity. The standard Yin Yang symbol is like the pre-heaven configuration with the light color, denoting heaven (Yang) above and the darker color, denoting earth (Yin) below. The practice of Tai Ji Quan utilizes the post-heaven configuration when it requires that Qi sink down from above (heaven) and that energy rise from below (earth), integrating at the Dan Tian to create internal power for daily living and longevity. This relates to the Daoist concept that the highest order of human endeavor is being able to conduct heaven and earth energy for the benefit of all. Tai Ji Quan incorporates this principle in the practice.

The approach to Tai Ji Quan described in this book was passed down by six generations of Masters. With the knowledge gained from Master Liu and decades of studying this system, I am passing on my limited understanding to forge a bridge and help the reader gain additional insights into this wonderful art. It is my sincere hope that the information will help enthusiasts of this art to achieve even greater heights.

FOREWORD
Hao ShaoRu

AFTER PUBLISHING the original Wu Style Tai Ji Quan in 1963, I received many letters from readers near and far, and I was interviewed by many journalists. Tai Ji enthusiasts expressed their curiosity about the ancient Tai Ji Quan manuscripts presented in the book and were interested in my father's theory. Their desire to accurately understand the meaning behind these Tai Ji Quan classics and their theory deeply touched me.

Wu Style Tai Ji Quan was published over 20 years ago. Due to the time constraints imposed by the publishing deadline, I was only able to introduce the movements of the form as the primary focus, and the descriptions are basic. In addition, the descriptions in the *Tai Ji Quan Classic* are expressed in generalities and utilize specialized terminology that is only suitable for use as a reference by advanced practitioners who have studied the subject in depth. For beginners and those who have not studied, it will appear to be impenetrable and abstract.

Based on the needs of the general audience, I accepted the People's Sports Publishing House's invitation to write another book that focuses on Tai Ji Quan's principles. I hope that this book will popularize the Wu Style Tai Ji Quan concepts and allow enthusiasts to learn and grasp them.

THIS BOOK CONSISTS OF
SIX DIFFERENT SECTIONS:

1. Chapter One contains a detailed description of the Yin Yang theory of Tai Ji Quan, an explanation of the meaning of the name Tai Ji Quan, and other key points.

2. Chapter Two contains a detailed description of Wu Style Tai Ji Quan's basic characteristics, the Body Principles, and the necessary learning process and steps to master this martial art.

3. Chapter Three contains a detailed description of the inner workings of Wu Style Tai Ji Quan practice, the basic principles and the practice guidelines for the form. There is a detailed and systematic explanation and discussion of the concepts of Intention and Force, Spaciousness, Relaxation, Roundness and Liveliness, Methods of Folding, Methods of Transformation, Three Insubstantial Embracing One Substantial, Five Bows, and Tai Ji Quan breathing.

4. Chapter Four uses figure drawings and written descriptions for a detailed explanation of Wu Style Tai Ji Quan form and the accompanying Body Principles.

5. Chapter Five presents a detailed description of the unique Wu Style Tai Ji Quan Striking Hands skill, as well as its basic practice methods and the relationship between form and Striking Hands practice. There is a theoretical discussion of "Leading to Emptiness, Borrow Strength to Strike Back" and its skill requirements. Finally, there are

the explanations of the intriguing Four Characters Secret Formula.

6. Chapter Six contains selections from the Tai Ji Quan Classic.

Wu Style Tai Ji Quan is also called Hao Style Tai Ji Quan and dates from the era of the Qing Dynasty XianFeng Emperor (1851-1861). It was introduced by Mr. Wu YuXiang[1] and has been taught for 130 years, with five generations of succession.

Mr. Wu passed the skill on to his nephew Li YiYu[2] and later passed it on to my grandfather, Hao WeiZhen who was his neighbor. Later, the Tai Ji Quan skills taught by Wu and Li were passed down and continued by the Hao family. Since the Hao family were able to carry on the tradition and expand on it and transmit it to others for several generations, over time it was also called Hao Style Tai Ji Quan.

My Grandfather's given name was He. His self-chosen name was WeiZhen (1849-1920). He followed Mr. Li, studying over many decades. He never stopped studying until Mr. Li passed away and thus was able to capture the essence of the Wu and Li family styles of Tai Ji Quan and become very skillful. He eventually passed the skills on to my father.

My father's given name was WenGui. His self-chosen name was YueRu (1877-1935). He began his studies with my grandfather when he was young. He also went to a school operated by Mr. Li and studied Chinese literature. When my

1. Wu YuXiang's given name is HeQing; his self-chosen name is YuXiang. HeBei province, YongNian county, Qing Dynasty Xiucai scholar rank, 1812-1880.

2 Li YiYu's given name is JingLun. His self-chosen name is YiYu, HeBei province, YongNian county, Qing Dynasty Juren scholar rank, 1832-1892.

grandfather was learning Tai Ji Quan from Mr. Li, my father often observed the teachings from the sideline. Through many years of observation and self-discovery, he was able to understand the subtleties before he reached maturity and learned the Tai Ji Quan skills in depth.

I was influenced by my family and their interests and background and began to study Tai Ji Quan with my grandfather and father when I was young. In time, with my father's guidance, I began to enjoy Tai Ji Quan and then developed a passion for it. By the age of fifteen, I had already acquired the habit of practicing Tai Ji Quan daily. So far, three successive generations of the Hao family have carried on the Wu and Li family Tai Ji Quan tradition, which has continued for over 100 years.

Tai Ji Quan contains martial techniques. It is also an art that requires skill. It is a creation of the rich and varied Chinese culture. Its theory and applications can be researched and used in a wide variety of areas.

It is my hope that I can assist in the propagation of Tai Ji Quan. If this book can benefit readers, I will be very happy! I hope to share the enjoyment of the knowledge of Wu Style Tai Ji Quan with all who study it.

There is no end to this art. My skills are limited. If there is anything in this book that is not adequate, please let me know.

Hao ShaoRu

Tai Ji Foundations

武式太極拳

CHAPTER ONE
THEORY OF TAI JI QUAN

CONCEPT OF TAI JI QUAN

TAI JI QUAN is a crystallization of Chinese wisdom and culture, a refined martial art based on a profound philosophy. If the practitioner first understands the deeper meaning of the name Tai Ji Quan, the direction of study will be clearer.

What is Tai Ji Quan? Simply put, Tai Ji refers to the internal movement of the body's Qi. Quan refers to the external movements of the body. Tai Ji and Quan combine and unify the internal movements of the Qi that leads to external, physical movements of the body. Using the energetics of Tai Ji to control Quan's movement is Tai Ji Quan. If there is only external movement (Quan) without the internal movement of Qi (Tai Ji), it can only be called a Quan exercise, not Tai Ji Quan. Thus, the practice of Tai Ji Quan must be the result of combining the internal and the external.

Tai Ji Quan is the application of an ancient Chinese philosophical concept to a martial art, which is why many people call it a philosophical martial art. Using Tai Ji in its name reflects its connection to the ancient philosophical concept of Tai Ji.

The theory of Tai Ji Quan requires that whether going forward or backward, turning to the left or to the right, with every motion the form of the accompanying Qi space (氣勢) must be full and complete without any imbalances. The name Tai Ji refers to the philosophical understanding of the embodiment of forces that are opposing and yet complementary.

Tai Ji Quan requires that each movement be composed of two sides which are opposing but can unify in their essence. By using intention, one can manifest highly coordinated, extraordinarily intricate and artistic movements. Tai Ji Quan, therefore, is an art more than just a technique.

The practitioner must know the significance of the name Tai Ji Quan and its relationship to the philosophical construct and methods of its motion. From this foundation, and by analyzing its theories, one can master its intricacies and methods.

Finally, the practitioner must be prepared and have the intention to study Tai Ji Quan as an art form from the very beginning. Thinking of it in purely technical terms is not useful for learning and mastering Tai Ji Quan.

YIN AND YANG THEORY OF TAI JI QUAN

The original meaning of Yin and Yang was taken from the observation of how the sun lights an object. When facing the sun, the front side is Yang, and the back side is Yin. The Ancients believed that Tai Ji is the foundation of the universe, separating into two: Yin and Yang Qi. The Tai Ji diagram is used to illustrate this cosmic phenomenon, indicating how opposing forces are one. (Diagram 1) Ancient philosophers looked at Yin and Yang as the two facets of all the material and societal world. The interaction of the two creates all the transformations and manifestations in nature. Therefore, exchanges between Yin and Yang form the rhythm of the cosmos. Tai Ji Quan uses this understanding to theorize, summarize and guide the study of this martial art. It demands that our intention and our body follow this oppositional yet complementary method for their movements. Yin and Yang therefore are the soul of Tai Ji Quan.

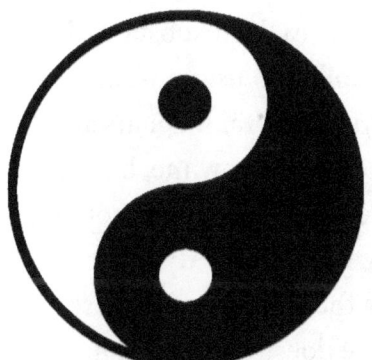

Tai Ji Diagram 1

As human beings, we wish all things would reach a successful conclusion. This is the meaning of round and full (圓滿). Being round and full means being complete and balanced. Tai Ji Quan requires that the energetic form be round and full, without corners or sharp angles, so there is no opening to be taken advantage of. Thus, each movement must contain the opposing forces of Yin and Yang. As the movement commences, the two are simultaneously acting and transforming, so that Yin and Yang are always where they should be, becoming the rhythm of Tai Ji motion.

The meaning at the heart of the art of Tai Ji Quan is this: As the physical form changes, one's Yin is never exposed to others; others can only touch Yang and never reach Yin. This is like the sunlight shining on an object. Yin will never be exposed to the sunlight.

How can Yin and Yang achieve internal power generation? It is by understanding and using the idea of substantial and insubstantial. Yin is substantial, substantial is Yin; Yang is insubstantial, insubstantial is Yang. Used correctly, the opponent only touches the insubstantial and never gets to the substantial. The ability to use substantial and insubstantial is an intriguing mystery of Tai Ji Quan's art. It can lead to a state in which others do not know me, but I know others. Thus, I can control others and others cannot control me. How Tai Ji Quan utilizes the endless dynamics of Yin and Yang to control others is the subtlety of this art. If one doesn't know Yin and Yang, one doesn't know Tai Ji.

Wu Ji and Tai Ji:
The Separation and Unification of Yin and Yang

Tai Ji arises from Wu Ji, the mother of Yin and Yang. This is the beginning of Wang ZongYue's classic treatise on Tai Ji Quan and explains very clearly that Tai Ji arises from Wu Ji. However, what is Wu Ji? Why does Tai Ji arise from Wu Ji?

Wu Ji represents the stillness of things, where there is no separation of Yin and Yang. Tai Ji represents the motion of things containing Yin and Yang Qi. Stillness and motion are in opposition. Therefore, Yin and Yang come from nothingness to something, meaning from Wu Ji to Tai Ji. In Wu Ji, Yin and Yang are united, not separated.

Tai Ji Quan starts from stillness. Before beginning its specialized motion, while the body is still and contains the potential for motion, there must be the feeling of fluidity and fullness. The body must be unified in preparation for movement, like a balloon (diagram 2). When the body reaches this potential, subsequent movement can be separated to Yin and Yang, creating Tai Ji Jin (勁). If the body of the practitioner is disjointed, even though there is intention for movement, the body cannot coordinate to create the potential for motion. The body cannot be engaged fully, and thus Tai Ji motion cannot commence. This type of movement is external, disordered and partial. The practitioner cannot move as one, coordinating the internal and the external. Therefore, without Wu Ji in readiness, there is no room for the birth of Tai Ji.

Wu Ji Diagram 2

The art of Tai Ji Quan arises from the fact that the transformations of Yin and Yang can manifest in limitless variations. Starting from stillness to motion (from Wu Ji to Tai Ji), then from motion to stillness (from Tai Ji to Wu Ji), stillness and motion are constantly transforming. Each movement from Wu Ji creates Tai Ji, separating to Yin and Yang Qi. Each stillness comes from Tai Ji back to Wu Ji, uniting Yin and Yang Qi. This is why it is said that in motion it separates, and in stillness it unites. This is the concept of Tai Ji Quan movement.

YIN AND YANG:
OPPOSING AND COMPLEMENTARY

Yin and Yang describe the two sides of how a movement which is oppositional comes about. If there are no opposing forces, then each side will lose the meaning of its own existence. For instance, insubstantial versus substantial, external form versus internal form, energy form versus spirit, flexible versus firm, motion versus stillness, all are opposing. The opposing forces of Yin and Yang exist only because of their oppositional reliance on and relationship with each other. Therefore, Yin and Yang are two sides that are in opposition, yet they can integrate to form movements.

Tai Ji Quan movements occur only when Yin and Yang are opposing and complementary. This is the fuel that provides energy for Tai Ji Quan as an art.

If one seeks to know how Yin and Yang are opposing and complementary, first one needs to know how to distinguish and integrate Yin and Yang.

Distinguishing Yin and Yang

Tai Ji Quan uses internal form as Yin and external form as Yang. Spirit is Yin, energy form is Yang; firm is Yin, flexible is Yang; stillness is Yin, motion is Yang. Stillness alludes to a calm heart, a relaxed spirit and a quiet body that is neither frozen nor stiff. What is above is Yang, what is below is Yin. What is in the front is Yang, what is behind is Yin. As to left and right, the determination of Yin and Yang must be made according to the actual situation, following the principle of Yin and Yang to decide. Even though Tai Ji Quan's movement and its relationship to Yin and Yang is complex, it does have a basic guiding theory and objective rules.

Yin and Yang are the two opposing sides of Tai Ji Quan movement. Internal versus external is another representation of the opposing nature of Yin and Yang. If there is internal there must be external. External motion is the following of others. Internal motion is based on self. In motion, the heart is calm, so that in movement there is stillness. This way, the movement will be tranquil. It is Qi that is in motion, which in turn powers the physical form. Qi is divided into Yin and Yang. Yin is spirit being attentive; Yang is the vibrant Qi preparing to move. Through Yin and Yang Qi, Tai Ji Quan found the wellspring for its motion. Gathering it will not deplete it. Using it will not weaken it. Tai Ji Jin is flexible and also firm. If it is too flexible, it will not have a structure; if it is too firm, it will become stiff. If Yin and Yang are not distinguished, it is called double weighting. Double weighting uses the natural inclination for physical movement. It does not provide room to be nimble or flexible. The resulting motion will be stiff and clumsy. Therefore, double weighting causes stagnation.

While distinguishing the Yin from the Yang, one must also notice the proportional difference between Yin and Yang. When Yin and Yang are equal, balance will be achieved. The pertinent sayings are "Stand like a balance (scale)," and "Not retreating and not opposing." When Yin and Yang are not equal, it creates an imbalance causing Jin not to be able to form properly and creating the effect of retreating or opposing. This is called "off balance, one must follow." (This "follow" is not the same as following others to gain strength; rather, it is falling off center). When one achieves Yin and Yang, both in opposition and harmony, then one can distinguish the Yin from the Yang.

Tai Ji Quan movement involves the whole body. Therefore, all segments of the body must have Yin and Yang. Insubstantial and substantial exist everywhere. At the same time, the oppositional energy of Yin and Yang must occur simultaneously in all places. This is the meaning of "Tai Ji is the whole body, and the whole body is Tai Ji."

Integration of Yin and Yang

When the practitioner can distinguish Yin from Yang, they will be able to work with them in unison. This is called the integration of Yin and Yang.

Internal and external form are in opposition, but at the same time they are in relationship, never abandoning each other. Therefore, only when internal and external motion are able to unify can Jin power, created by the internal workings of insubstantial and substantial energy, be embodied in every movement. Let's take another example of Spirit and Qi space: Spirit must support Qi space, and at the same time Qi space must surround Spirit. This way the Qi space is lively, and Spirit will not disperse. Internally, Spirit is gathered, and externally it feels comfortable. Spirit is firm; energy is soft. In softness there is firmness. This way it is flexible but has structure, is firm but not obvious. The Jin that is created will become elastic and springlike.

In summary, Yin and Yang must be able to mutually contain, diffuse, and permeate each other and have the ability to unite and work together to reach the place where "Yang does not leave Yin. Yin does not abandon Yang. Yin and Yang are integrated."

TRANSFORMATION OF YIN AND YANG

When Yin and Yang can work together effectively while simultaneously being opposed and unified, it implies that there is a path where the energy is able to transform, where insubstantial can become substantial and substantial can become insubstantial. Once insubstantial and substantial can transform, the wonderous ability to shift and adapt to the opponent's force will provide insight and a path to higher skills, finally reaching the miraculous Tai Ji realms of "Others do not know me, but I know others. I control others but others cannot overcome me."

To rearrange properly, it does not matter if one is practicing form or Striking Hands. Adjustments of the insubstantial and substantial must be made based on the actual circumstances. While practicing form, depending on how the postures are moving, the insubstantial and substantial must interchange. While performing Striking Hands, depending on the opponent's insubstantiality and substantiality, one must adjust one's own insubstantiality and substantiality. For example, while practicing the Left Lan Zha Yi form, the left hand is higher and forward and is insubstantial; the right hand is below and behind and is substantial; the left leg is forward and is insubstantial, and the right leg is behind and is substantial.

While using Left Lan Zha Yi form for Striking Hands practice, since it is not known where the opponent's force might make contact, one must rearrange the insubstantiality and substantiality of the contact point based on where the opponent's force is landing. Wherever the contact point, Yin and Yang need to separate at that point, then stick, connect, adhere, and follow, tracking the opponent to control him. If going from Left Lan Zha Yi to a different posture, for the energy to transform, the insubstantial and substantial of the up and down, left and right and front and back must adjust based on the footwork and the arm movement. For example, if moving to Right Lan Zha Yi, the right hand is on top and in front and becomes insubstantial. The left hand is below and behind and becomes substantial. The right leg is in front and becomes insubstantial, and the left leg is in back and becomes substantial.

The transformation of insubstantial and substantial occurs internally, not externally. Going from the internal and manifesting to the external is the meaning of "Jin is internally exchanged." Once the methods of transformation are learned, and one becomes skillful, insubstantial and substantial can adjust freely. It does not matter whether one is going forward or backward, or turning to the left or to the right, power can be expressed effectively. This is how Tai Ji Quan's art enters the realm of the mysterious and miraculous.

UNDERSTANDING TAI JI THEORY
Commonality and Particularity

Tai Ji Quan movements are unique, but at the same time they have much in common with other forms of movement. The primary difference is that the movements of Tai Ji Quan are both internal (based on the movement of Qi) and external (physical). These movements embody the integration, opposition and transformation inherent in the theory of Yin and Yang.

Tai Ji Quan's theory of Yin and Yang stems from conclusions drawn from the actual experiences of Tai Ji Quan practitioners during practice. In order to fully comprehend the theory of Tai Ji Quan, as well as to master the art of Tai Ji Quan, one must understand its particularities as well as its irregularities. Only then may one understand its commonality with all physical movement.

Importance of Practice:
The Path to Learning the Yin Yang Theory of Tai Ji Quan

The theory upon which Tai Ji Quan is based is the foundation of the actual physical movements. It is the compass for actualizing the practice, and the only path to understanding the art of Tai Ji Quan. But, of course, these theories were developed from the generalizations and summaries of other people's experience. Therefore, for the reader, this poses a certain amount of abstractness and indirectness.

Obviously, it is impossible when one begins the study of Tai Ji Quan to immediately know and understand the theories. Only through diligent practice and constant reflection on Tai Ji Quan's theory will a higher and deeper knowing develop. Only when the practitioner develops a certain amount of feeling for Tai Ji Quan's movement is it possible to gain insight into Tai Ji Quan's principles and theories.

The study of Tai Ji Quan needs theory to guide its practice. Practice also needs to accurately reflect the theories, principles and guidelines. When all are present, one can master the art of Tai Ji Quan. Only when one learns how to apply the principles in the practice, is it possible to digest the abstract and indirect nature of those theories, and to make the knowledge one's own. At that point theory and practice become one. This is the fundamental way to gain mastery of the art of Tai Ji Quan.

Finally, theories provide guidelines for accurate practice. At the same time the indispensable element for understanding the theories is continuous, diligent practice.

CHAPTER TWO
FEATURES OF WU STYLE
TAI JI QUAN

DISTINGUISHING ATTRIBUTES

WU STYLE TAI JI QUAN is also called Hao Style Tai Ji Quan. This style follows the principles of Tai Ji Quan faithfully and conforms to all its theories and methods. Its special characteristics are: Use Tai Ji (internal form) as the central focus, and use internal Jin and mind-intention to deploy Qi. Practice unifying Jing (精), Qi (氣) and Shen (神) as one[1].

The Tai Ji Quan form passed down by Wu YuXiang and Li YiYu originally had 53 Forms. My father, based on my grandfather's understanding, converted the 53 Forms, with each form emphasizing the four principles of initiate, engage, express and converge throughout, and expanded it to today's 96 Forms.

Because the individual Wu Style Tai Ji Quan forms utilize the principles of initiate, engage, express and converge throughout, all movements are constructed based on this sequence.

Wu Style Tai Ji Quan not only uses initiate, engage, express and converge throughout, but the body, arm

---

1 Please read Introduction for explanations of Jing, Qi and Shen.

and footwork also all follow Tai Ji Quan's principles faithfully. Whether going forward or retreating, turning left or turning right, maintaining a centered torso is the foundation. With centering the tailbone as a prerequisite, and emphasizing going from the internal to the external, the footwork meticulously follows the principle of separating the insubstantial and the substantial. When transferring from insubstantial to substantial, the emphasis is on using internal strength and not physical strength. This means not leaning the body back and forth or left and right or rising and falling (except when going low or jumping) to accomplish the task. It places high muscular demands on the waist and legs, making it a strenuous exercise. The hands are mainly used in an open vertical position, and do not extend over the toe. The left and right arms stay on their respective sides of the body and should not casually reach across. The entire form practice places the emphasis on the body, arms and footwork coordinating organically with the integration of the internal and external. In other words, internal energy transformation directs external motion.

The unique features of the art of Wu Style Tai Ji Quan are adapting to the opponent's force and borrowing the opponent's strength to use against them. The saying "Lead to emptiness. Four ounces redirect one thousand pounds" refers to the interaction of intention and Qi. By focusing on using internal power while being inconspicuous, and transforming without the opponent knowing, ("Others do not know me. I know others"), the miraculous realm of "Others are controlled by me, but I am not controlled by others" is achieved.

WU STYLE TAI JI QUAN'S BODY PRINCIPLES

Importance of the Body Principles

Tai Ji Quan, as a specialized human movement, has unique requirements and guidelines that form the Body Principles for the torso, arms and legs.

The art of Tai Ji Quan is built on the foundation of the Body Principles. The Body Principles are the key link for organizing the internal form to generate internal power. Therefore, the body, arm and footwork must follow the theories of Tai Ji Quan as the basis for their motion and must work in cooperation to reach the goal of using internal energy to direct external form.

My father, after careful analysis, summarized those body, arm and footwork principles as the 13 Wu Style Tai Ji Quan Body Principles. They are: relax and open the chest; open the back; round the buttocks; protect the stomach; suspend the head; suspend the pelvis; relax the shoulder; sink the elbow; center the tailbone; movement in stillness; express Jin; Qi Sinks to the Dan Tian; and distinguish the insubstantial from the substantial. Therefore, when the Body Principles are mentioned in Tai Ji Quan, it can be understood as a general expression for the torso, arm and footwork.

Due to the importance of the Body Principles for Tai Ji Quan practice, generations of Wu Style Tai Ji Quan practitioners regard the teaching and practice of the Body Principles as a central element for learning.

The requirements of the Body Principles in Wu Style Tai Ji Quan are precise and detailed. The practitioner must practice diligently for a period of time before accurately understanding how the principles of body, arm and footwork can function naturally and organically, so that each movement can meet the proper guidelines.

Body Principles (Hao YueRu)

1. What is Relax and Open the Chest?

涵胸 Relax and Open the Chest: The chest is above the heart. Do not push it outward. The chest must relax so that the Qi can travel downward. Both shoulders should round slightly forward and converge, so that heart intention can deploy Qi.

2. What is Open the Back?

拔背 Open the Back: Open between the shoulder blades and energetically float up. The shoulders need to be nimble and agile. Do not lower the head.

3. What is Round the Buttocks?

裹襠 Round the Buttocks: Feel energy at the back of the knee. The legs have the sensation of coming together and feel like one. It is necessary to distinguish the insubstantial from the substantial.

4. What is Protect the Stomach?

護肫 Protect the Stomach: The lower rib cage feels like it is coming together slightly. There is a sensation of gathering from below and converging forward from above. Internally, one feels comfortable and at ease.

5. What is Suspend the Head?

提頂 Suspend the Head: The head and neck stay centered. Do not lower the head or pull it upward. Spirit rises to the top of the head to suspend the whole body.

6. What is Suspend the Pelvis?

吊襠 Suspend the Pelvis: Feel the force at the upper thigh. The buttocks move forward so that the lower abdomen has a sense of lifting.

7. What is Relax the Shoulder?

鬆肩 Relax the Shoulder: Use mind-intention to open the shoulder. Qi sinks down. The intention of stillness needs to be part of it.

8. What is Sink the Elbow?

沉肘 Sink the Elbow: Use intention to deploy Qi at the elbow. The wrist needs to be flexible and agile. The elbow needs to have a downward intention.

9. What is Movement in Stillness?

騰挪 Movement in Stillness (prepare to move): Forming the intention to move, the body is at the ready right before movement commences.

10. What is Express Jin?

閃戰 Express Jin: The body, hands, waist and legs are connected and follow each other, acting as one, moving outward like releasing an arrow. Fast as lightening, it cannot be stopped.

11. What is Center the Tailbone?

尾閭中正 Center the Tailbone: Feel strength at the upper thigh with the buttocks gathered forward. The tailbone shifts forward energetically, upholding and embracing the Dan Tian.

12. What is Qi Sinks to the Dan Tian?

氣沉丹田 Qi Sinks to the Dan Tian: Once the tailbone is centered, the chest is relaxed and open, the stomach is protected, the shoulders are relaxed and the pelvis is suspended, intention can send the Qi to the abdomen so that it will not rise.

13. What is Distinguishing the Insubstantial and the Substantial?

虛實分清 Distinguishing the Insubstantial and the Substantial: One must be able to distinguish insubstantial and substantial between the two legs. The insubstantial leg is not completely empty. The substantial foot, which touches the ground, needs to have the energy of movement in stillness (be prepared to move). The energy of movement in stillness means that the insubstantial leg has a pulling or attracting sensation with the chest, otherwise, it is off-center. Substantial does not mean holding firm. Spirit focuses on the upper thigh of the substantial leg to support the entire body with the intention of lifting. If one cannot distinguish the insubstantial and substantial, it is called double weighting.

PROCESS OF LEARNING WU STYLE TAI JI QUAN

When studying Wu Style Tai Ji Quan, one must carefully follow Tai Ji Quan's theory to direct one's own practice. Grasping and understanding the essence of Tai Ji Quan is a step-by-step process. Thus, from familiarity gradually comes knowing. From knowing, one eventually reaches the realm of the intuitive. Without persistent practice this cannot be attained.

The Three Levels of Learning Tai Ji Quan

FIRST LEVEL
LEARNING THE FORM

There is a common saying: "All tall buildings start at the foundation." Learning Tai Ji Quan is like constructing a tall building. The foundation needs to be strong so it can rise high. Studying the form is the first step in learning Tai Ji Quan. When one first learns calligraphy, one must follow the rules for every stroke. The same is true for learning Tai Ji Quan. Place importance on the correctness and accuracy of each posture. To improve, grasp the pattern and direction of each movement in the whole form. Strive to make each posture precise. To build a solid foundation for the form, keep the body centered at all times. One mistake to avoid is hurrying to learn the intricacies before learning the form properly. When one tries to skip around rather than learn step-by-step, it is easy to go off course.

SECOND LEVEL
LEARNING THE BODY PRINCIPLES

Proficiency of form provides the foundation from which to learn the Body Principles. Because the Body Principles are the foundation for the internal forms, they are a critical step for acquiring skill in Tai Ji Quan. Learning Wu Style Tai Ji Quan without the foundation of the Body Principles is impossible.

Of course, comprehending the Body Principles all at once is not possible. One should choose one or two basic principles to initiate the practice. Once they are understood, add more until you can grasp all of them and link them together as a whole.

From the foundation of the body being centered, studying the Body Principles should begin with centering the tailbone. Next, proceed to relaxing and opening the chest, opening the back, rounding the buttocks, protecting the stomach, suspending the head, suspending the pelvis, relaxing the shoulder, sinking the elbow, distinguishing the insubstantial from the substantial, and so forth, learning them one after another. Next, one must seek to collect the Qi to the lower back (lumbar region) and cause Qi to surround the waist. When the Qi from the lower back can surround the waist, the body has a master. When the body has a master, the body, arm and footwork can connect together in unity. The whole body, bones and muscles, are then able to coordinate and work efficiently together. From this point on, one begins to acquire the ability to use Qi for movements.

THIRD LEVEL
LEARNING JIN (INTERNAL POWER)

The essence of the art of Tai Ji Quan can be found in its proper application to human biodynamics. The creation of force does not arise externally but internally. These internal manifestations then transform into fascinating internal power. Thus, in everyday form practice, each movement must proceed from the internal to the external so that it is integrated.

When studying the use of internal power, one must understand how mind-intention, as well as the transformation, deployment and application of Qi, moves the body using internal form to direct external movement.

In everyday practice, one must analyze and reflect upon the meaning of spaciousness, relaxation, roundness and liveliness. The Qi space needs to be full and the Spirit vibrant, so that it is possible to work on the ability to support all eight directions. For Qi to move and fill all corners, the body must be connected, not disjointed. Before one can use mind-intention to direct and employ Qi, one must be able to distinguish and separate mind-intention and Qi. Qi must be nourished and gathered without the body rising. The abdomen must open and relax. Qi from the spine region must pass through the tailbone, move forward and turn upward to the Dan Tian. The Qi space can then become lively. Upon reaching this level, one can use mind-intention to deploy the Qi to activate Jin in the whole body. Every movement needs to be initiated with mind-intention. Qi moves, and next the body moves, so that all three, mind-intention, Qi and Quan become one. Starting from the external to the internal, from unfamiliarity to full awareness of the Qi, slowly the whole body feels like a balloon. It makes no difference if one is moving forward or backward or turning left or right, the Qi space is full and round.

When one reaches this level, internal and external are one. It is neither rough nor precise. If it exists, it exists. If it is gone, it is gone and forgotten. Every move is natural and intuitive, with no thought as to why one's hand is moving or one's foot is dancing.

CHAPTER THREE
INNER WORKINGS OF WU STYLE TAI JI QUAN PRACTICE

意與力

YI AND LI (INTENTION AND FORCE)

WHAT IS YI? How is Yi used? Why do we use Yi and not Li? What is the meaning of Li? As practitioners, we must learn to thoroughly understand Yi and Li and be able to distinguish between them to improve.

The principles of Tai Ji Quan require that one use intention and not force. Whether one is practicing form or Striking Hands, every movement is directed by intention rather than muscular force and utilizes intention for its subtlety and effectiveness.

The ability to apply intention to physical movement is achieved through an understanding of the principles of Tai Ji Quan. Following deep reflection on how to apply intention to physical movements, one will naturally use intention along with a corresponding perceptual awareness to carry out movements according to the Tai Ji Quan principles. During practice, when feelings, thoughts, and imagination are used in combination, the result is called Yi. In essence, this practice utilizes the central nervous system, functioning in a highly aware manner, to generate movements. Once the practice is mature, the movement becomes a natural reflection of our intention.

Learning the Tai Ji Quan principles requires mental awareness of bodily sensations as part of the learning process. Careful study leads one to utilize this mental awareness to direct one's movement during practice. Eventually, the learner is able to use both thought and kinesthetic sensation to create this type of movement. The ability of Tai Ji Quan to direct the body for very detailed and complex motions is a result of a highly developed human consciousness.

In the saying "Use intention and not force," the word force refers to using muscular tension as feedback, as opposed to mind-intention. Using only muscular sensation results in movements initiated without using one's full awareness, and indicates that one is not able to distinguish between mind-intention and Qi, or between insubstantial and substantial. Muscular tension is simple, direct and without variation, and easily exposes one's intent. As a result, others can take advantage of you.

The reason that Tai Ji Quan requires the use of mind-intention and not force is that by using intention to train the body one can convert one's natural habits of movement, which rely on muscular sensation, into the new, subtle and ingenious internal power called Jin. For the beginner, who does not understand Tai Ji Quan principles clearly and has difficulty matching intention and Qi sensation, the result is that the body is not able to move properly. This problem cannot be avoided at the start. However, with diligent, thoughtful practice, while using intention as part of each movement, practitioners gradually will be able to transition from using excessive muscular force to the proper use of intention. With persistent practice, one naturally can reach the stage when mind-intention initiates, Qi activates, and physical form then follows. Mind-intention, Qi and Quan will begin to harmonize. Eventually one's consciousness can direct every part of the body, reaching the realm of "If it exists, it exists. If it is gone, it is gone." Everything follows the heart's intent.

空鬆圓活

SPACIOUSNESS, RELAXATION, ROUNDNESS AND LIVELINESS

In higher level practice, the physical body will feel expansive, as if it is in suspension. The entire body will feel like a giant ball. At this point one can move the Qi at will, and movements will be felt as lively, like a wheel. To reach this level, one must understand spaciousness, relaxation, roundness and liveliness.

Spaciousness, relaxation, roundness and liveliness are only four words, but to understand their deeper meaning is not a simple task. Every single word has its own methods and usage, but at the same time, they are related. When they work together, one will discover their wonders.

Spaciousness and Relaxation

Tai Ji Quan is not simply relaxed motion. If one only pursues relaxation but not spaciousness, one cannot enter a higher level. To make the muscles relax and the joints open is easy, but to achieve spaciousness is difficult. Therefore, one must understand and work on spaciousness.

In Tai Ji Quan movements, one needs to distinguish between spaciousness and relaxation, but at the same time one cannot forego either. These two aspects are opposing but are also mutually dependent. If one simply pursues relaxation without spaciousness, one will be loose, collapsed and dispersed. However, if one only pursues spaciousness without relaxation, one will only get a mental illusion of expansiveness without substance. This type of movement is also not useful. The practice of Tai Ji Quan must unify both the mental and the physical aspects of the movement and not just be simple imagination. Therefore, if one desires spaciousness, there must be relaxation; if one desires relaxation, there must be spaciousness. They work together in an organic manner to bring Qi to one's movements. This is one of the big difficulties in learning Tai Ji Quan. Only pursuing one or the other will not honor the duality at the core of Tai Ji Quan.

Spaciousness and relaxation must be carefully studied during daily practice. For the muscles and bones to relax and open, there must be the intention of spaciousness; for spaciousness, there must be thoughts of relaxation. With persistent practice, the opposing natures of spaciousness and relaxation can be reconciled. Once this step is taken, there is hope of reaching the higher realms of Tai Ji Quan.

Before any movement commences, most beginners experience anxiety. Because of this, the muscles and joints are unnaturally tight, which makes movement difficult. To make comfortable movements, thoughts must be relaxed and the principle of using intention and not muscular force must be kept in mind until the heart is calm and the body is at ease. Eventually the feeling of spaciousness with intention rising, and relaxation with Qi sinking will be present. Muscles and bones will seem to separate. At this point one enters the realm of roundness and liveliness.

Roundness and Liveliness

To reach the realm of liveliness, the Qi space must be round and full. More roundness implies more liveliness. Roundness is the basis for liveliness. The saying goes, "Round is alive, and angular is stagnant." To enter the realm of roundness and liveliness, one must be able to control one's Qi space (氣勢) and support the eight directions[1] (八面支撐).

Qi space formation is dependent upon one's internal practice. The size of the Qi space is one way of determining the depth of one's practice. The larger the Qi space, the deeper the practice. This is the meaning of "Tai Ji Quan is not based on physical form but on Qi space. It is not external, it is internal." As a practitioner, one must not underestimate the importance of this. The basis for Qi is the ability to understand and express spaciousness and relaxation. Roundness and liveliness cannot be separated from first having spaciousness and relaxation. If one has not reached a certain level of spaciousness and relaxation, roundness and liveliness cannot be attained. Once the requirement of roundness and liveliness has been fulfilled, one will understand the wonders and full extent of spaciousness and relaxation.

If the requirement of Qi is to be round and full, that means Qi must occupy a certain space and not disperse

---

1 The eight directions refers to all the surrounding Qi space.

into nothingness. If it is contained in a space, it must have a center and a circumference. During one's practice, one must imagine a Qi space that can be controlled by intention, using the waist as the center. In every movement, one must respect this space. No movement can go beyond its boundary, but at the same time one must be connected to the boundary. This way the space will not be uneven or bumpy, and it can become full.

When the boundary is farther from the center, bigger Qi space is required to occupy it. Qi must be supported by Spirit. Spirit needs to fill and support all eight directions. This way Qi will be full and will not weaken. Qi must also surround Spirit so that Spirit is not exposed. When one achieves this, Qi is round and full, and Spirit can become vibrant.

How does Spirit support all eight directions? Using the waist as the center, one must employ intention to create the eight directions for support. All eight directions must be equal for Qi to be round and full. If the eight directions are uneven, the Qi space will not be smooth and balanced.

During regular practice, one must pay careful attention to the Qi space and its eight directional supports. In the beginning, most students are not able to understand and express this. Thus, one must be attentive during practice. As time goes on, one will be able to express it in the body. Openness is expansion of the Qi using the waist as the center and reaching outward in all eight directions. Convergence is contraction of the Qi using the waist as the center for gathering all eight directions. It does not matter if the Qi is expanding or contracting, the boundary of the Qi space is passive. It is the waist that initiates and commands.

If one comprehends the above and can use it in the practice, Qi space will not be chaotic, and it will not matter if one is going forward or backward or turning left or right. In every movement the Qi space will be full and round. When this happens, as one moves the arms, Qi will move in a correspondingly rounded manner between the arms and chest.

If one has roundness, one will have liveliness. The energy of liveliness is internal and not external. When the external follows the internal, internal power will not be fractured. As movement is derived and initiated from the motion of Qi and not from external motion, one's body is unified. At this point, Qi naturally flows through the body and can freely transform in all eight directions and turn at will. Thus, as intention initiates, the Qi will be able to follow, and intention and Qi will respond naturally to any stimulus. When reaching this realm, it does not matter if one is going forward or backward, to the left or to the right, going up or going down, bending or straightening, expanding or contracting. In every movement the Qi can move freely. One will have found liveliness. This is the meaning of "Qi is like the wheel. Lively as the wheel."

折疊之術

METHODS OF FOLDING

Folding is the way to combine and unite opposing energies. The process is based on the idea that if there is up, there is down; if there is down, there is up; if there is a front, there is a back; if there is a back, there is a front; if there is right, there is left; if there is left, there is right. Folding is not only included in the movement of internal energies, it is also the inner structure of the Body Principles.

Folding expresses itself during the motions of internal energy. When the intention is going up, there is a simultaneous intention of going down. Up intention and down intention should be equal. When intention goes down farther, the up intention should follow by going higher. It does not matter if it is forward or backward, to the left or to the right, the energy must be equal. This is the method of folding.

With the Body Principles, folding requires the separation of the four direct and the four cross alignments. In the four direct alignments, the shoulders should square up with the hips. The left shoulder should match directly with the left hip, and the right shoulder must match up with the right hip. The two up and down energies must match and be equal. The four cross alignments are the left shoulder matching with the right hip and the right shoulder matching with the left hip. The cross energies also must match and be equal.

Once you have achieved the four direct and the four cross folding requirements, it is possible to use the spine as the center, with matching energy on the left and right sides of the body. Once this happens, the body can maintain its balance and does not move randomly. Compliance with each of the Body Principles can come to fruition and manifest.

轉換之法

METHODS OF TRANSFORMATION

Energy transformation in Tai Ji Quan uses a unique method of converting energy between Yin and Yang and insubstantial and substantial. Once one understands this concept and is able to utilize it, one has built the equivalent of a bridge to master Tai Ji Quan.

To understand how they transform, the relationship of Yin and Yang and insubstantial and substantial need to be clearly grasped. The key point is the two eyes of the waist. The term eyes of the waist refers to the two dimples by either side of the spine at the base of the lower back near the waist. When transforming, the intention is at the waist. When turning to the left, the left waist eye pulls up slightly, and the right waist eye slides under and lifts the left waist eye. The left chest should become insubstantial. When turning to the right, the right waist eye pulls up slightly and the left waist eye slides under and lifts the right waist eye. The right chest becomes insubstantial. When stepping to the left, the left waist eye pulls up slightly, and the right waist eye slides under and lifts the left waist eye. Spirit should focus on the right upper thigh of the substantial leg and use the energy of preparing to move for the left leg to step forward. When stepping to the right, the right waist eye pulls slightly up and the left waist eye slides under and lifts the right waist eye. Spirit should focus on the left upper thigh of the substantial leg and use the energy of preparing to move for the right leg to step forward. When stepping back with the left leg, the left waist eye pulls up slightly and the right waist eye slides under and lifts the left waist eye. Spirit focuses on the right upper thigh of the substantial leg and uses the energy of preparing to move for the left leg to step back. When stepping back with the right leg, the right waist eye pulls up slightly, the left waist eye slides under and lifts the right waist eye. Spirit focuses on the left upper thigh of the substantial leg and uses the energy of preparing to move for the right leg to step back. When one waist eye moves up, the other moves down. One is substantial and the other is insubstantial. The substantial slides under and lifts the insubstantial. The insubstantial and substantial must stay connected and mutually dependent. Yin cannot be separated from Yang, and Yang cannot be separated from Yin. Yin and Yang must work together so that the energy can transform. The insubstantial can transform to substantial; the substantial can transform to insubstantial. It is important to remember that Jin is transformed internally. The transformation of substantial and insubstantial is accomplished internally not externally. Only from the internal can energy express to the outside. When the energies are transformed internally, there will be no outward manifestation, so that the realm of "others do not know me, and I know others" can be reached. Physical form follows the activation of intention. Footwork follows the internal body transformation from internal to external.

三虛包一實

THREE INSUBSTANTIAL EMBRACING ONE SUBSTANTIAL

Three Embracing One is a distinctive method used by Wu Style Tai Ji Quan to understand and use the relationship between insubstantial and substantial. In Tai Ji Quan movement, insubstantial and substantial exist in and apply to every part of the body. How insubstantial and substantial are reflected in Tai Ji Quan movement is very complex. However, there are principles to follow. For instance, if up is insubstantial, down is substantial; if front is insubstantial, back is substantial; if left is insubstantial, right is substantial; if right is insubstantial, left is substantial. In the relationship between the arms and the legs, if both arms are up, above is insubstantial and the legs below are substantial. In the relationship between the two legs, if the left leg is insubstantial, the right leg is substantial; if the right leg is insubstantial, the left leg is substantial. Consequently, the relationship between the arms and the legs is three insubstantial embracing one substantial. If the left leg is substantial, the right leg and both arms are insubstantial; if the right leg is substantial, the left leg and both arms are insubstantial. Insubstantial means having the energy of preparing to move. Substantial is attentiveness of the Spirit. Spirit is substantial and stays within and hidden. Qi space is insubstantial and must embrace and surround the Spirit. "Three Insubstantial Embracing One Substantial" means using intention so that the two arms and the insubstantial leg are embracing the one substantial leg.

Tai Ji Quan requires Qi to embrace the Spirit, so that the Spirit can be contained within. In return the Spirit must support the Qi, so that the Qi space can be full. In learning Three Embracing the One, one must pay careful attention to how intention uses Spirit to support the Qi space. If used properly, in insubstantial there is substantial, and in substantial there is insubstantial. The substantial is hidden and the insubstantial is not loose, collapsed or dispersed, thus following the principles of Tai Ji Quan.

五张弓

FIVE BOWS

Tai Ji Quan has a saying: "Gather Jin like pulling a bow. Release Jin like releasing an arrow."

Tai Ji Quan bases its theory on the characteristics of human physiology and structure and divides the body into five bows: The torso is the main bow, and the two arms and two legs are complementary bows. In gathering and releasing, the four complementary bows must work under the governance of the main bow, moving organically and systematically so the Jin of the entire body can be energized at the same time. However, a person and a bow are different in form and quality. In practicing Tai Ji Quan, intention is used to create the effect of pulling the bow and releasing the arrow, which enables one to borrow another person's force and use it against them.

Main Bow

Wu Style Tai Ji Quan uses the spinal column as the main bow. The upper spine and the tailbone are the bow tips, and the lower back (Gate of Life 命門), around the lower curvature of the spine is the grip (center) of the bow. The upper end of the main bow connects to the arms and the lower end connects to the legs. The lower back is the center that connects to the four complementary bows.

Practitioners, when practicing the form, must use the lower back as the center dividing line. What is above needs to conform to the energy principle of opening the back; what is below the tailbone must lift the Dan Tian (lower abdomen) to achieve suspension of the pelvis. At the same time, intention creates a sense of connection between the collarbone area and the Dan Tian, like the string on a bow, while at the lower back (grip of the bow), the Qi must converge and collect. This way the main bow will create the "Jin of Gathering," which is similar to the springlike energy of a bow. The gathering movement creates the power to release the arrow.

When the main bow is gathering and releasing, neither push the lower back backward nor hunch the upper back. The lower back, as the grip of the bow, cannot move backward. If the lower back moves backward, it will lose its centering position, creating an imbalance and becoming lopsided. If so, the Qi cannot converge to be collected and will lose its ability to lead. Instead, to stay centered, the lower back must have the intention of moving forward, thus having the ability to govern the whole body and to create the effect of pulling the bow and releasing the arrow. This is an internal motion. The abdomen is not pushing outward physically. The saying "Gather Jin like pulling a bow, release Jin like releasing an arrow" refers to intention, not physical form. Pulling the bow uses intention to replace physical form or force. Jin is not created by changing the physical shape. It is internal not external.

Arm Bows

There are two arm bows. The hand and shoulder are the tips of the bows, and the elbows are the grips of the bows. In gathering and releasing, the two hands and both shoulders must have the intention of attracting and connecting, like bows with the bowstring on. The grips of the bows, the two elbows, need to have a sensation of sinking.

Leg Bows

There are two leg bows. The hip and foot are the tips of the bows, and the knees are the grips of the bows. In gathering and releasing, both hip and foot must have the intention of attracting and connecting, like a bow with the bowstring on. As the grips of the bows, the two knees need to have the intention of rising.

Five Bows as One

If one wants to "gather Jin like pulling a bow, and release Jin like releasing an Arrow," all five bows must be used together, and function and connect as one. Functioning as one means that when one bow pulls, all the rest of the bows must pull. In releasing all must release. When one bow stops, all bows must stop. In connecting as one, the main bow is the commander. The entire body's Jin behaves like a single bow, from the foot to the leg, to the waist and reaching the fingers, united and energized as one. When it is energized as one, Jin can concentrate and be directed to one targeted place. Gathering is like an in-breath, and releasing is like an out-breath. Just as an in-breath can naturally seize and pick up a person, an out-breath naturally sinks down and releases a person. This is the ingenious aspect of the five bows working as one.

Therefore, while practicing the forms, during each movement one must ask oneself if all five bows are present. The five bows must connect as one and be controlled at the waist. The bows must be springlike for them to gather and release. Practicing form is like Striking Hands, Striking Hands is like practicing form. The principle is the same. The critical element is gathering. If the bow can be pulled effectively, Jin can be expressed efficiently.

太極拳的呼吸即是[蓄發，開合，收放]

TAI JI QUAN BREATHING CONSISTS OF GATHER AND RELEASE, OPEN AND CONVERGE, AND RECEIVE AND DISCHARGE.

Tai Ji Quan breathing uses the metaphor of breathing to describe the concept of "leading to emptiness, borrowing force to strike back." Tai Ji Quan breathing is different in quality, usage and substance from natural breathing. However, these two different methods of breathing occur simultaneously during practice. If we do not carefully differentiate between them, it is very easy to confuse the two and reach the wrong conclusion. Many practitioners lose their way due to this misunderstanding.

When one practices Tai Ji Quan, one must first understand natural breathing and Tai Ji Quan breathing. By being able to distinguish and separate them, it is possible that, with practice, one can understand Tai Ji Quan breathing.

Natural breath supports life by gathering oxygen and releasing carbon dioxide. This system requires many organs such as the nose, mouth, throat, trachea and lungs to complete. It goes on night and day with a set frequency and depth, has a tempo, works autonomously, and does not require conscious control. Tai Ji Quan breathing, instead, uses conscious control to direct the flow of Qi. This type of breathing occurs only while we are performing Tai Ji Quan. The reason breath is used as a metaphor to describe this activity is that the movement of Qi in this martial art is similar to the movement of air in natural breathing. Gathering the opponent's force, just like breathing in air, and then converting that force and releasing it back, striking the opponent using Jin, is like breathing air out. Breathing in the force and then transforming it and breathing it out as Jin follows an objective movement pattern. In-breath is contracting the Qi space inward to store it as Jin in the body. This is the gathering process. Out-breath is expanding the Qi space outward and discharging the Jin that is stored. This is the release process.

The saying is: "In-breath is convergence and gathering; out-breath is opening and releasing. To converge is to receive. To open is to discharge." Therefore, Tai Ji Quan breathing means gathering and releasing, opening and converging, receiving and discharging. It is very different from natural breathing.

The practitioner can use conscious control and subtle movement changes for "leading to emptiness, borrowing the force to strike back." The ability to use this type of specialized breathing requires the intention to train in a disciplined manner to accomplish this task. If there is no conscientious practice, there will be no Tai Ji Quan breathing.

In Tai Ji Quan practice, there are many sayings such as "Qi Sinks to Dan Tian," "Moving the Qi," and "Qi Rising." The experience of this kind of Qi implies that when one has reached a certain level of practice, one is able to consciously feel a particular sensation that is not due to breathing air. Do not let this Qi sensation be confused with breathing in and out from the nose and mouth.

73

In the process of learning Tai Ji Quan, natural breathing will change following the physical needs of the body. In this process both breathing patterns will simultaneously exist. Tai Ji Quan requires that the whole body move as one. One's natural inclination is to use force, but this force must be transformed to intention-based Jin. The Body Principles are the key to this transformation. These principles form the basis and provide a systematic way of training one's internal energy to create Jin. Once the principle of "Qi Sinks to the Dan Tian" is mastered, the center of gravity will be naturally lowered. Natural breathing will follow and become deep breathing. This change is a result of the practice of Tai Ji Quan and is different from other intention-based deep breathing practices.

Tai Ji Quan practice can convert natural breathing to a deep breathing pattern, causing many practitioners to develop an erroneous understanding of the relationship between Qi Sinks to the Dan Tian and natural breathing. They often make the mistake of doing abdominal breathing, either pushing out, or contracting the lower abdominal muscle to simulate mastery of the principle that Qi Sinks to the Dan Tian. The reality of the matter is not that simple. Tai Ji Quan practice does not allow any pushing in or out or contracting of any abdominal area. Mastery of Qi Sinks to the Dan Tian must be achieved through conscious effort that organically unites one's internal energy. To manifest this deep breathing phenomenon, one must be able to master the principles of center the tailbone, open the chest, protect the stomach, relax the shoulder, suspend the pelvis, and other Body Principles. Next one must be able to nurture and gather and fulfill the requirement that Qi Sinks to the Dan Tian. Consequently, if one can do deep breathing, it is not necessarily equivalent to the Tai Ji Quan principle of Qi Sinks to the Dan Tian. However, if one can master the principle of Qi Sinks to the Dan Tian, one's breathing will be naturally deep. Typical deep abdominal breathing practice does not conform to the Body Principles and therefore will naturally not get the same benefits as a result.

Qi Sinks to the Dan Tian is a special requirement of Tai Ji Quan. It is not a requirement of natural breathing. The deep breathing pattern that occurs from Tai Ji Quan practice is due to the actualization of the Body Principles, which does not require conscious control on the part of the practitioner. However, to master these Body Principles does require conscious intention.

Regular breathing will naturally adapt to one's physical needs at any given moment, regardless of the situation. Breathing is instinctual and regulates itself without conscious effort. While gathering Jin in Tai Ji Quan, one will naturally take an in-breath. While releasing Jin, one will naturally use an out-breath. This syncing of two types of breathing is a natural occurrence with the action of Open and Converge and Gather and Release. However, one's natural breathing frequency cannot fulfill Tai Ji Quan's deep and long Gather and Release oxygen requirement. Therefore, the two breathing frequencies are not always in lock step. The normal breathing process and frequency is based on physical demand and the associated oxygen requirement. It is also limited by lung capacity. When one inhales, one cannot exhale, and when one exhales, one cannot inhale.

The Tai Ji Quan breathing process and frequency is based on the needs of Tai Ji Quan movement: Not only can one inhale and inhale, and exhale and exhale, one can also simultaneously inhale while exhaling ("In Convergence There is Opening"), and exhale while inhaling ("In Opening There is Convergence"). This is like a long, winding river or the ocean, never ending. One can take from it without depleting it and use it without exhausting it. Therefore, if one tries other methods to control breathing frequency to master open and converge, not only can one not acquire Tai Ji Quan's art, it might not be good for one's health.

In Tai Ji Quan movement, it is important to follow the Body Principles precisely. These principles are the guarantees for mastery of the art of Tai Ji Quan. The breathing pattern will naturally shift with the practice of these principles. When the body becomes spacious and open, Qi can naturally sink down. As the chest opens wider, the lung capacity will increase, and thus the breath will be deeper. This all occurs naturally and does not require special practice to change the regular breathing frequency or depth. Tai Ji Quan movement does not require monitoring one's breathing and does not require natural breathing to direct Tai Ji Quan's Open and Converge movement. Careful attention must be devoted to the ways of Tai Ji Quan breathing during practice.

WU STYLE TAI JI QUAN PRACTICE GUIDELINES (HAO YUERU)

Essence of the Practice:

手，眼，身，步，精，氣，神

Hand, Eye, Body Principle, Footwork,
Jing, Qi and Spirit

Without being scattered, the hands and arms must have a vibrant Qi Space with the energy of preparing to move. Both shoulders should be open and spacious, without the feeling of muscular tension. The arms do not have a preferred direction. It does not matter if they are moving up or down, or extending or retracting, as long as there is a corresponding intention. When does the intention initiate and when does the arm arrive? This is what is meant by heart-mind and arms working in harmony (得心應手). The sequence of the energy of preparing to move is: have Intention, move Qi, concentrate Spirit. Use intention to move Qi. With persistent practice, one will become efficient. As efficiency improves, it becomes more spontaneous. As practice matures, it becomes intuitive and natural. By following this logic, one will understand the subtlety of Spirit.

Spirit is gathered in the eye; the eye is the seedling of the heart; the heart arises from intention. When the intent is to move in a direction, the eye will focus on that direction, and then the body will also point to that direction. Thus, with a turn of the eye, the whole body turns. In stillness there is movement, and in movement there is stillness. All comes from the gathering of Spirit.

According to the Body Principles, one must first seek to center the tailbone. To be centered, the tailbone must move forward. At the same time, one must have the energy of protecting the stomach. Without it one cannot have the energy to straighten the tailbone and there is no power to direct the body. When the intention is going toward a direction, the tailbone will point to the same direction. Turns and changes happen between the two waist eyes. Turning left means the left waist eye pulls slightly upwards, using the right waist eye to lift the left waist eye. Turning right means the right waist eye pulls slightly upwards, using the left waist eye to lift the right waist eye. This way the tailbone will find the center naturally. Overall, each of the Body Principles must be correctly applied. In combination they become one united Body Principle. When any Body Principle is off, the whole body is off. Therefore, the Body Principles must always be correct. It does not matter how circumstances change; it is difficult to go beyond the Body Principles.

This is what it means to distinguish the substantial and the insubstantial in the footwork. Insubstantial does not mean absence of force. Internally there is the energy of preparing to move. Substantial does not mean exerting force. The Spirit is concentrated. Preparing to move is called insubstantial. In insubstantial there must be substantial. Spirit is called substantial. In substantial there is insubstantial. Insubstantial and substantial, substantial and insubstantial, this is the intent.

起承開合

Initiate, Engage, Express and Converge

When practicing Tai Ji form, each form has four movements: The first movement is initiate (like the first step of left Lan Zha Yi); the second movement is engage (the second step of left Lan Zha Yi); the third movement is express, which is equivalent to projection (the third step of left Lan Zha Yi); the fourth movement is converge, which is equivalent to gathering, which means storing (the fourth step of left Lan Zha Yi). None of the movements are rigid. In expressing, continue to express, and in converging, continue to converge. This is the meaning of not retreating and not opposing (不丟 不頂). Everything is just right.

Core of the Form Practice

When practicing form, the heart must be calm. Calming the heart enables the mind to concentrate. When the mind is concentrated, it is possible to focus on practice. When one is able to focus on practice, one is able to conform each movement to Tai Ji Quan's requirements and eventually one will be able to move the body accordingly. This way, awareness is used in the highest order. Every movement is directed by intention without being scattered. Eventually one can concentrate fully. At the same time, Spirit is centered and the body is calm. To progress from intention to physical movement requires persistent practice. When intention activates the Qi and the Qi moves the body, intention, Qi and form practice can harmonize as one. For this reason, the heart must be calm.

To nourish and gather the Qi without having it rise, the Body Principles must be practiced and thoroughly understood. Qi sinks down means the shoulders need to be relaxed and open. If the shoulders are not relaxed, Qi cannot sink down. At the same time, sinking the Qi also requires relaxing the chest. If the chest is not relaxed and collected, Qi cannot sink to the Dan Tian. When relaxing the chest, one must be careful not to collapse the chest inward. The requirements of protecting the stomach and suspension of the pelvis must be accompanied by relaxing the chest. Without protecting the stomach, the abdominal area cannot be relaxed and full, Qi cannot radiate, and the tailbone cannot stand. Without suspension of the pelvis, Qi cannot be gathered and nourished. Once these Body Principles are achieved, the Qi will not rise. This shows why the Body Principles must be diligently practiced.

The energy of preparing to move must be present and extend from the arms to the fingers. To relax and open the shoulder, the intention must be below the elbow. For Qi to reach the fingers, sinking the elbow must have the intention below the palm. The two arms and both sides of the chest must feel connected. The arms are directed by each side of the chest and have the sensation of being lively and round. When this requirement is achieved, the motion of the arms will not be scattered, and the chest can transform energy.

The two legs must be able to gather strength. If the legs desire to gather strength, the hip cannot lean to the right or left relying on muscle tension. Instead use intention to open the hip joint area vertically (open the Qua). For the two legs to be connected as one, it is very important to distinguish the substantial from the insubstantial between the legs while at the same time rounding the buttocks. Rounding the buttocks is the result of intention and is not physical. When stepping left, the left hip pulls up slightly, and the right hip shifts under and lifts the left hip. Stepping to the right, the right hip pulls up slightly and the left hip shifts under and lifts the right hip.

Substantial is not rigid. Instead, Spirit is concentrated. Insubstantial is not an absence of force. Instead, it has the energy of preparing to move. Within insubstantial there is substantial, and within substantial there is insubstantial. Jin is changed internally. Step as if walking on thin ice, then the footwork will be light, nimble and secure.

When practicing, every movement must be composed and stable, while keeping light and moving freely. Upon acquiring this ability, the body's movements will no longer be scattered. Spirit is fully aware, but Spirit cannot externalize. Spirit is focused but also centered. This is what it means to "internalize the Spirit while externally at ease" [内固精神，外示安逸]. The entire body, upper and lower, and the internal and the external must be connected and yet remain open. The art of moving the Qi, expressing the Jin, transforming, and opening and converging can be found internally not externally. The practitioner must take note: If a movement is not directed by internal form, it cannot be called Tai Ji Quan.

While practicing the form, one must be able to distinguish four actions, initiate, engage, express and converge, in every movement. Ask which action is activated as the movement commences and find the flavor and use of each. Between each action there is continuity. Each action flows to the other smoothly without stagnation. In expressing, there is convergence, and in convergence there is expressing.

Form practice is a way of learning how to know oneself. In each movement ask if any requirements are missing or realized. Practicing this way, self-correcting the form and making improvements, is the way to achieve the highest skill in Tai Ji Quan.

One important point is that while practicing, the forms must be done slowly enough to know if the proper requirements are being fulfilled. To feel the interaction between intention and Qi, the pace of the form must be slow.

Tai Ji Quan does not require fast movements, rather it is about learning to transform intention and Qi and understanding the internal workings of the Tai Ji Quan skills. Thus, "when others are fast, they cannot get ahead of my intention; when others are strong, they cannot compare to my collected Qi." However, the pace of the form cannot be too slow. When it is too slow, it is difficult for the Qi to be continuous, and stagnation will be the result.

CHAPTER FOUR
WU STYLE
TAI JI QUAN FORMS

EXPLANATION OF FORM SEQUENCE
AND BODY PRINCIPLES

IN WU STYLE Tai Ji Quan all movement, from beginning to end, is based on four energetic components: initiate, engage, express and converge (起，承，開，合). Together these components form the basis of a sequence of Movements. For example, the second form, Left Lan Zha Yi, consists of four Movements displayed in sequence in the following Four Diagrams: Diagram A (initiate), Diagram B (engage), Diagram C (express) and Diagram D (converge).

In between each sequence, there may appear to be a slight pause, however when Jin stops, Intention and Qi must continue without interruption. Therefore, during form practice, the energy should not be disrupted.

Each form, as detailed above in Left Lan Zha Yi, combines four or more Movements to create a sequence. However, there are places where as few as two and as many as five forms are combined to create a sequence as is the case when the fourth form, Single Whip and the fifth form, Lift Hand are combined and form the four Movements to make a complete sequence.

Illustrations of Sequence with Body Principles
for Left Lan Zha Yi

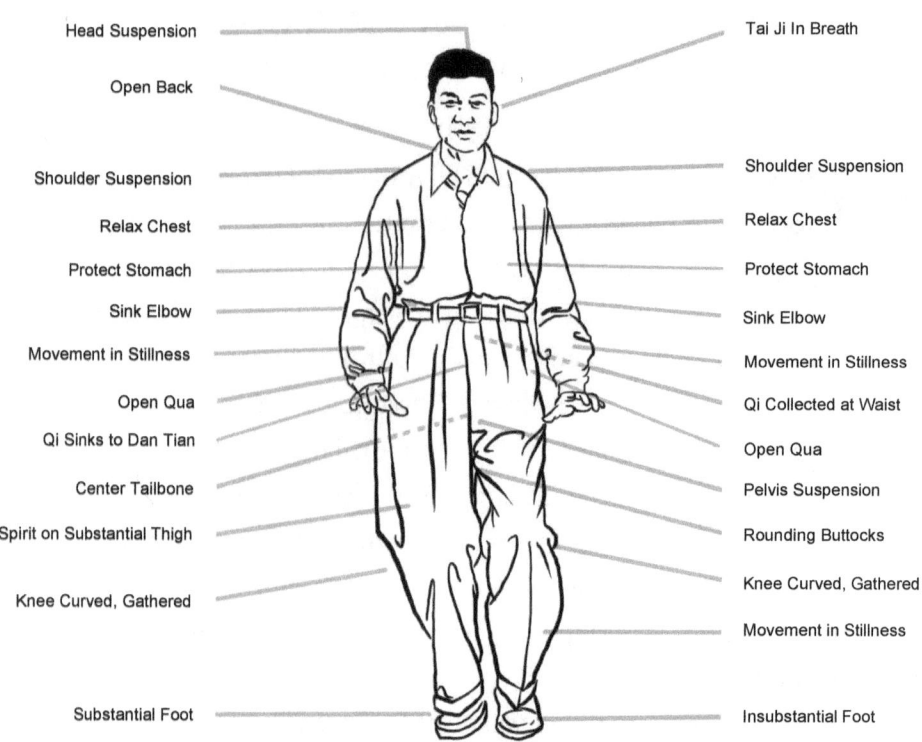

Head Suspension

Open Back

Shoulder Suspension

Relax Chest

Protect Stomach

Sink Elbow

Movement in Stillness

Open Qua

Qi Sinks to Dan Tian

Center Tailbone

Spirit on Substantial Thigh

Knee Curved, Gathered

Substantial Foot

Tai Ji In Breath

Shoulder Suspension

Relax Chest

Protect Stomach

Sink Elbow

Movement in Stillness

Qi Collected at Waist

Open Qua

Pelvis Suspension

Rounding Buttocks

Knee Curved, Gathered

Movement in Stillness

Insubstantial Foot

A. INITIATE

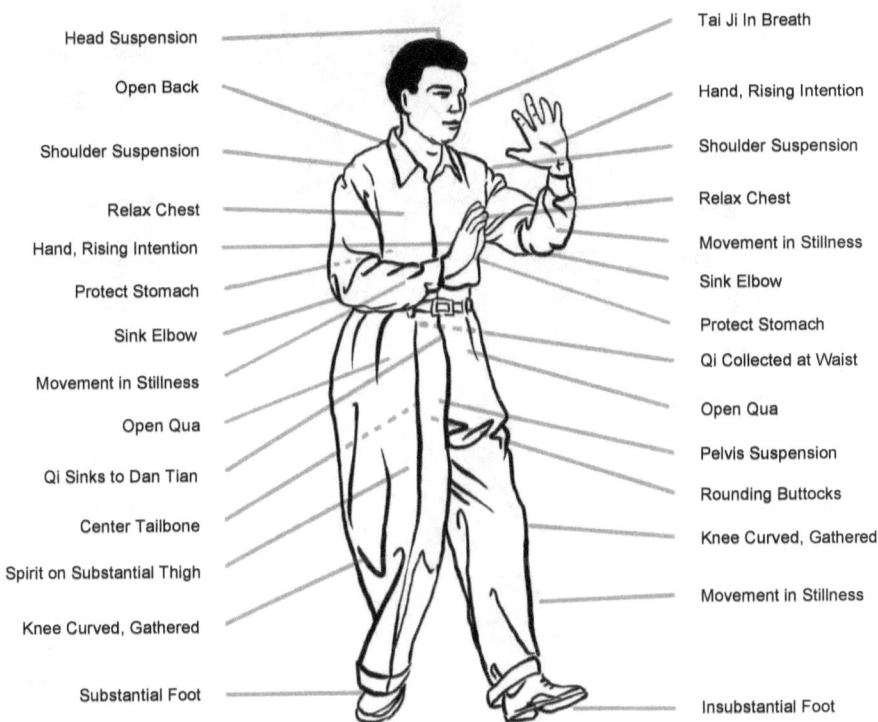

Head Suspension

Open Back

Shoulder Suspension

Relax Chest

Hand, Rising Intention

Protect Stomach

Sink Elbow

Movement in Stillness

Open Qua

Qi Sinks to Dan Tian

Center Tailbone

Spirit on Substantial Thigh

Knee Curved, Gathered

Substantial Foot

Tai Ji In Breath

Hand, Rising Intention

Shoulder Suspension

Relax Chest

Movement in Stillness

Sink Elbow

Protect Stomach

Qi Collected at Waist

Open Qua

Pelvis Suspension

Rounding Buttocks

Knee Curved, Gathered

Movement in Stillness

Insubstantial Foot

B. ENGAGE

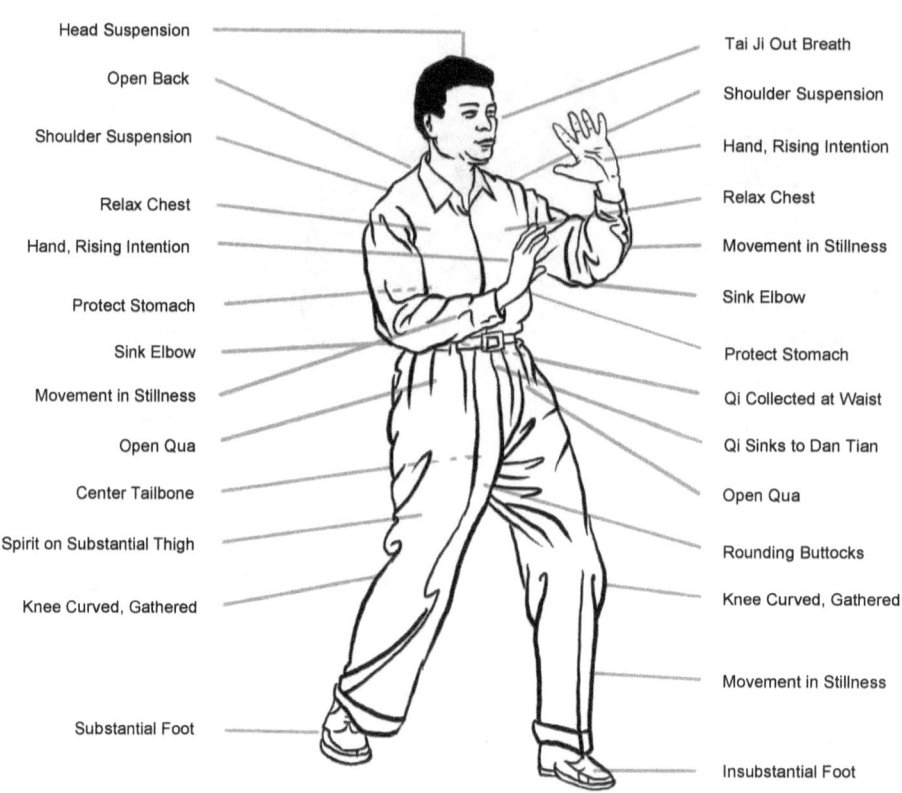

Head Suspension

Open Back

Shoulder Suspension

Relax Chest

Hand, Rising Intention

Protect Stomach

Sink Elbow

Movement in Stillness

Open Qua

Center Tailbone

Spirit on Substantial Thigh

Knee Curved, Gathered

Substantial Foot

Tai Ji Out Breath

Shoulder Suspension

Hand, Rising Intention

Relax Chest

Movement in Stillness

Sink Elbow

Protect Stomach

Qi Collected at Waist

Qi Sinks to Dan Tian

Open Qua

Rounding Buttocks

Knee Curved, Gathered

Movement in Stillness

Insubstantial Foot

C. Express

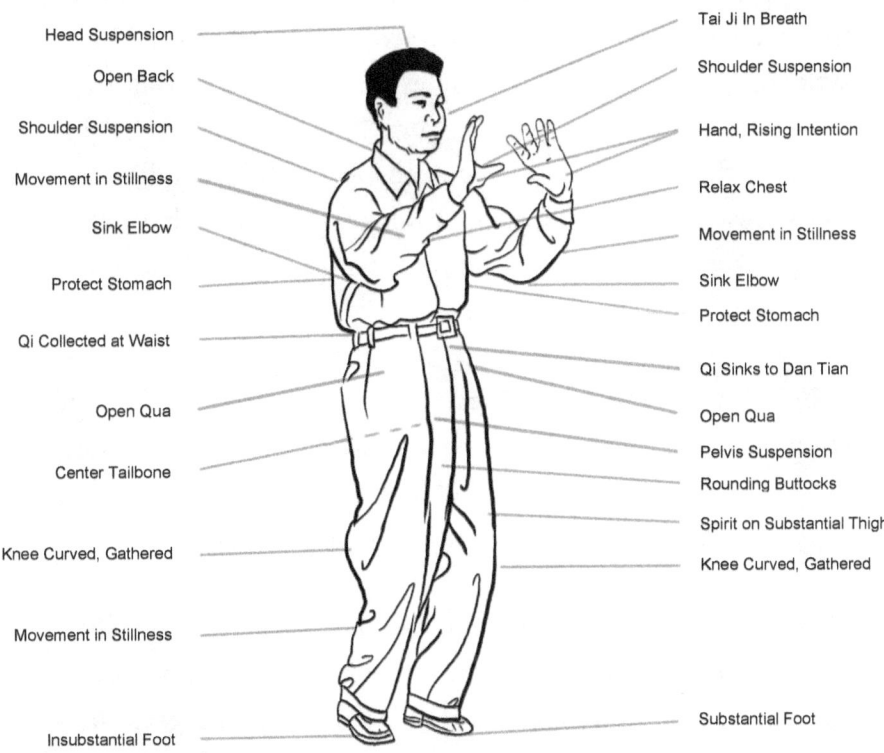

Head Suspension

Open Back

Shoulder Suspension

Movement in Stillness

Sink Elbow

Protect Stomach

Qi Collected at Waist

Open Qua

Center Tailbone

Knee Curved, Gathered

Movement in Stillness

Insubstantial Foot

Tai Ji In Breath

Shoulder Suspension

Hand, Rising Intention

Relax Chest

Movement in Stillness

Sink Elbow

Protect Stomach

Qi Sinks to Dan Tian

Open Qua

Pelvis Suspension

Rounding Buttocks

Spirit on Substantial Thigh

Knee Curved, Gathered

Substantial Foot

D. CONVERGE

DEFINITION OF BODY PRINCIPLES
IN THE ILLUSTRATION

The labels that accompany the diagrams refer to the Body Principles illustrated in each of the sequences of diagrams that are the basis for the body, arm and footwork of Wu style Tai Ji Quan. These principles form the basis of all the movements and are very important. Therefore, even though some of them have been discussed before, to facilitate the study, research and comprehension of this style, they will be repeated here with additional expanded Body Principle requirements with explanations.

涵胸 **Relax and Open the Chest:** The chest is above the heart. Do not push it outward. The chest must relax so that the Qi can go downward. Both shoulders should round slightly forward and converge, so that heart-intention can deploy Qi.

拔背 **Open the Back:** Separate at the waist (around the MingMen/kidney area) with the intention that the upper area will rise up between the shoulder blades. Open energetically and float up. The shoulders need to be nimble and agile. Do not lower the head.

裹襠 **Rounding the Buttocks:** Feel energy at the back of the knee. The two legs have the sensation of being one and connected. Do not push the legs together physically. It is necessary to distinguish the substantial from the insubstantial.

護肫 **Protecting the Stomach:** The lower rib cage feels as if it is coming together slightly. There is a sensation of gathering from below and converging forward from above. Internally one feels comfortable and at ease.

提頂 **Suspending the Head:** The head and neck stay centered. Do not lower the head or pull it upward. Spirit rises to the top to suspend the whole body.

吊襠 **Suspending the Pelvis:** Feel energy at the upper thigh. The buttocks move forward. The waist has downward intention. The tailbone has the intention of moving forward to hold the lower abdomen. The lower abdomen feels like it is uplifting.

鬆肩 **Relaxing the Shoulder:** Use mind-intention to open the shoulder. Qi sinks down. The intention of stillness needs to be part of it.

沉肘 **Sinking the Elbow:** Use intention to move the Qi at the elbow. The wrist needs to be flexible and agile. The elbow needs to have a downward intention.

騰挪 **Movement in Stillness (prepare to move):** Form the intention to move before moving so that the body is ready before movement commences.

尾閭正中 **Center the Tailbone:** Feel energy at the upper thigh. The buttocks move forward with the sensation of gathering inward. The tailbone shifts forward energetically, upholding and embracing the Dan Tian with the intention and sensation that the tailbone and C7 vertebra are in alignment.

氣沉丹田 **Qi Sinks to the Dan Tian:** Once the tailbone is centered and the chest is relaxed and open, protect the stomach. When the shoulders are relaxed, and the pelvis is suspended, intention can direct the Qi to the abdomen and the Qi will not rise.

虛實分清 **Distinguishing the Insubstantial and the Substantial:** One must be able to distinguish which leg is insubstantial and which leg is substantial. The insubstantial leg is not completely empty. The insubstantial foot, which touches the ground, needs to have the energy of movement in stillness (prepare to move). The energy of movement in stillness means that the insubstantial leg has a pulling or attracting sensation with the chest. Otherwise, it is off-center. Substantial does not mean holding firm. Spirit focuses on the upper thigh of the substantial leg to support the entire body with the intention of lifting. If one cannot distinguish the insubstantial and substantial, it is called double weighting.

腰脊斂氣 **Qi Collected at the Waist:** Use intention to create the sensation of the shoulders opening outward in a spacious and relaxed manner. Simultaneously there will be a sensation of gathering inward toward the spine. Next use intention to direct Qi to flow down the back and collect at the waist. When Qi collects at the waist, it can fill the waist. When Qi fills the waist, the waist can take command.

胯鬆直 **Open the Qua:** The hips should not tilt to the left or the right. They must not be tense. Using intention to open and straighten the hips in a relaxed manner allows the Qi to sink down and lets the two legs (thighs) gather strength.

膝曲蓄 **Knees Curved and Gathered:** It is necessary to be able to distinguish which leg is insubstantial and which is substantial. One must not be stiff or static. For the Jin to be pliable and springlike, it must be able to accumulate in a curve. Therefore, the legs should not be straight. At every point of the sequence (initiate, engage, express or converge) both knees must have a curve to store energy.

两手意向上升 **Two Hands With Rising Intention:** Energetically, both hands must rise while the base of the palm sinks down (Sitting the Wrist). The fingers have the intention of lengthening so Qi can move through the fingers. This is called rising intention.

WU STYLE TAI JI QUAN'S
96 FORM NAMES

1.	起勢	Begin
2.	左懶扎衣	Left Lan Zha Yi
3.	右懶扎衣	Right Lan Zha Yi
4.	單鞭	Single Whip
5.	提手上勢	Lift Hand
6.	白鵝亮翅	White Swan Spreads Wings
7.	摟膝拗步	Brush Knee Twist Step
8.	手揮琵琶	Play the Guitar
9.	摟膝拗步	Brush Knee Twist Step (2)
10.	手揮琵琶	Play the Guitar
11.	上步搬攬捶	Step Forward, Parry, Repulse and Punch
12.	如封似閉	Withdraw and Push
13.	抱虎推山	Carry Tiger, Push Mountain
14.	手揮琵琶	Play the Guitar
15.	右懶扎衣	Right Lan Zha Yi
16.	單鞭	Single Whip
17.	提手上勢	Lift Hand
18.	肘底看捶	Fist Under Elbow
19.	左倒攆猴	Left Repulse Monkey
20.	右倒攆猴	Right Repulse Monkey
21.	左倒攆猴	Left Repulse Monkey
22.	右倒攆猴	Right Repulse Monkey
23.	手揮琵琶	Play the Guitar
24.	白鵝亮翅	White Swan Spreads Wings
25.	摟膝拗步	Brush Knee Twist Step
26.	手揮琵琶	Play the Guitar

27.	按勢	Press Down
28.	青龍出水	Green Dragon Rises Out of Water
29.	翻身	Turn Around
30.	三甬背	Three Changing Backs
31.	單鞭	Single Whip
32.	下勢	Down Posture
33.	紜手	Cloud Hands (2)
34.	單鞭	Single Whip
35.	提手上勢	Lift Hand
36.	高探馬	High Pat on Horse
37.	左伏虎	Left Taming Tiger
38.	右起脚	Right Kick
39.	右伏虎	Right Taming Tiger
40.	左起脚	Left Kick
41.	轉身蹬腳	Turn Around and Left Heel Kick
42.	單鞭	Single Whip
43.	踐步打捶	Skip and Punch
44.	翻身二起	Turn, Double Rise
45.	披身伏虎	Step Back, Taming Tiger
46.	退步左踢脚	Step Back, Left Kick
47.	轉身右蹬腳	Turn Around and Right Heel Kick
48.	上步搬攬捶	Parry, Repulse and Punch
49.	如封似閉	Withdraw and Push
50.	抱虎推山	Carry Tiger, Push Mountain
51.	手揮琵琶	Play Guitar
52.	右懶扎衣	Right Lan Zha Yi
53.	斜單鞭	Diagonal Single Whip
54.	下勢	Down Posture

55.	野馬分鬃	Wild Horse Parts Mane (3)
56.	單鞭	Single Whip
57.	玉女穿梭	Fair Lady Weaves Shuttle (4)
58.	手揮琵琶	Play the Guitar
59.	右懶扎衣	Right Lan Zha Yi
60.	單鞭	Single Whip
61.	下勢	Down Posture
62.	紜手	Cloud Hands (2)
63.	單鞭	Single Whip
64.	下勢	Down Posture
65.	更雞獨立	Rooster Stands on One Leg (2)
66.	左倒攆猴	Left Repulse Monkey
67.	右倒攆猴	Right Repulse Monkey
68.	左倒攆猴	Left Repulse Monkey
69.	右倒攆猴	Right Repulse Monkey
70.	手揮琵琶	Play the Guitar
71.	白鵝亮翅	White Swan Spreads Wings
72.	摟膝拗步	Brush Knee Twist Step
73.	手揮琵琶	Play the Guitar
74.	按勢	Press Down
75.	青龍出水	Green Dragon Rises Out of Water
76.	翻身	Turn Around
77.	三甬背	Three Changing Backs
78.	單鞭	Single Whip
79.	下勢	Down Posture
80.	紜手	Cloud Hands (2)
81.	單鞭	Single Whip
82.	提手上勢	Lift Hand

83. 高探馬　　　High Pat on Horse
84. 對心掌　　　Heart Palm
85. 轉身十字擺蓮　Turn, Cross Lotus Kick
86. 上步指襠捶　Step Up, Low Punch
87. 跟步懶扎衣　Step Up, Right Lan Zha Yi
88. 單鞭　　　　Single Whip
89. 下勢　　　　Down Posture
90. 上步七星　　Step Up to the Seven Stars
91. 退步跨虎　　Step Back Over Tiger
92. 轉身雙擺蓮　Turn, Lotus Kick
93. 彎弓射虎　　Bend Bow Shoot Tiger
94. 雙抱捶　　　Double Punch
95. 手揮琵琶　　Play the Guitar
96. 收勢　　　　End

CLARIFICATIONS OF ILLUSTRATIONS, AND INDICATORS

The descriptions of each movement attempt to be as precise and concise as possible. Supplementary explanations describing the essence of each movement are included so the reader can grasp and understand the form accurately.

In Wu style Tai Ji Quan each movement either faces one of the four cardinal directions (south, north, east, or west) or one of the four intercardinal directions (southeast, southwest, northeast or northwest). A figure facing the reader is facing south.

In each figure the dashed lines represent the direction of movement of the left arm and leg, and the solid lines represent the direction of movement of the right arm and leg. The arrows at the end of the lines indicate the start of the direction of movement of the next figure.

If the description of the movement has already been given for a prior form, the figure will still be shown in sequence. However, the explanation of the movement will not be repeated.

To enhance the detailed understanding of the footwork, shadows are used to distinguish how the foot interfaces with the ground. There are four different ways the foot relates to the ground: the foot is flat on the ground, the heel touches the ground, the toe touches the ground, the foot is in the air. When the foot touches the ground, there is a shadow. If there is no shadow, the foot is in the air.

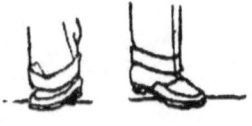 Whole Foot Touching Ground

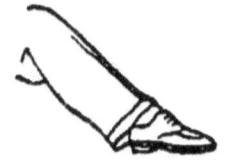 No Shadows When Foot Off Ground

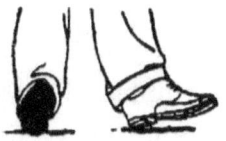 Heel Touching Ground

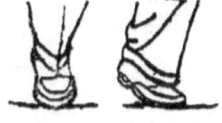 Toe Touching Ground

WU STYLE TAI JI FORMS
WITH EXPLANATIONS

1.Prepare to Begin (Figure 1)

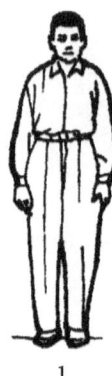

1

The two feet are together with the toes pointed slightly outward and with the heels one fist apart. Both knees are slightly bent and should never be straight. The two arms fall naturally at the sides. The eyes look forward. (Figure 1)

Key points: When standing with the two feet together, the body posture should be natural and at ease. Spirit is uplifted, without extraneous thoughts. The head is straight, and the chin is pulled slightly inward. Suspend the head insubstantially to lift the body. Relax and open both shoulders. Relax the abdominal area using the proper Body Principles: relax the chest, open the back, round the buttocks, protect the stomach, sink Qi to the Dan Tian and so forth.

The following descriptions include the 4 steps of a sequence. Movement 1 is initiate, 2 is engage, 3 is express and 4 is converge.

2. Left Lan Zha Yi (Figures 2-5)

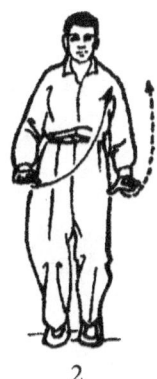

2

Movement 1:

Slightly bend both knees. The right leg is substantial, and the left leg is insubstantial. The left heel is up, with the toe touching the ground. At the same time, both arms are slightly bent. The arms rise forward and up and then lower next to the hips, with the backs of the hands facing up, and the fingers pointing forward and slightly curved and separated.(Figure 2)

Key points: While moving, the practitioner needs to keep the Body Principles in mind. When lowering the arms, the head must be suspended insubstantially to lift the body up. Once the legs start to move, it is necessary to clearly distinguish between the insubstantial and the substantial. The body must not lean. The two arms, when moving downward, need to have the feeling that the two shoulders are attracting and pulling them to complete the task. At the same time, when the arms are lowering, both elbows need to stay in front of the rib cage and have the sensation of sinking down, while simultaneously synchronizing harmoniously with the movements of the legs.

In the Wu Style Tai Ji form, in all the movements and postures, no matter if it is initiate, engage, express or converge, the arms and legs should not completely straighten. They need to have a certain amount of curvature. This discussion will not be repeated in the following descriptions.

Movement 2:
Look to the southeast. The body turns slightly to the left. With the turn, the left leg lifts, taking a step to the southeast. The heel touches the ground first with the toe pointing upward. The right leg is still substantial and the left is insubstantial. At the same time, both arms rise in front of the chest in the vertical palm position with the edge of the palms naturally facing forward. The vertical palm always has the edge of the palm facing forward. This instruction will not be repeated below. The left arm is ahead and above, at shoulder height. The right hand is behind and below at chest height. The head faces southeast (Figure 3).

Key points: The body should not turn excessively. When the arms are raised, they need to have the intention of gathering and leading the opponent's incoming force, while at the same time having the intention of lifting the left leg to step forward. The right leg needs to have Spirit concentrated and must support the movement of the left leg. Keep the body principles intact.

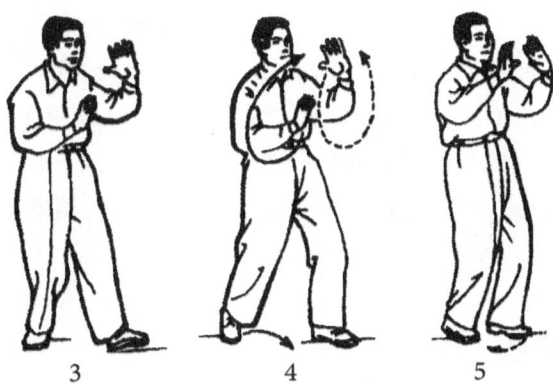

3　　　　　4　　　　　5

Movement 3:

The right heel pushes forward. The left leg shifts forward to form a curve and lands flat on the ground, and the body moves forward. The legs are still right substantial and left insubstantial. At the same time, the two vertical palms push forward slowly toward the southeast with the left arm at shoulder height. The right arm moves forward and slightly downward from the chest. The head faces southeast. (Figure 4)

Key points: Immediately before the right leg pushes, the two arms in front of the chest draw a curve from low to high. This is called leading, gathering and accumulating to express. Leading and gathering need to follow each other seamlessly with a forward intention. During express, the body cannot float up. In the Wu Style Tai Ji form, except when skipping and bending down, the body should not rise or sink. The upper and lower body need to coordinate, keeping the tailbone centered and maintaining the other Body Principles intact.

Movement 4:

Keep facing the same direction. Both arms, with vertical palms, sink down to the hip level and immediately separate to the left and right. They then rise in a curve with both vertical palms in front of the chest, as if pushing a ball. Both hands are at shoulder height. When the arms are just getting ready to rise, the legs transform to become left substantial and right insubstantial. As both arms rise, the right leg moves up next to the left leg, with the toe pointing to the ground. (Figure 5)

Key points: While both arms are moving downward, both shoulders should have the intention of attracting and pulling the arms, and both sides of the chest need to direct the movement of the arms. At the same time, both elbows should stay in front of the rib cage. The space between the upper arm and the chest needs to feel round and lively. Before the back leg starts to come up, the two legs should complete the transformation of insubstantial and substantial. While the back leg is moving up, the upper and lower body need to coordinate properly. The Body Principles apply.

3. Right Lan Zha Yi (Figures 6-9)

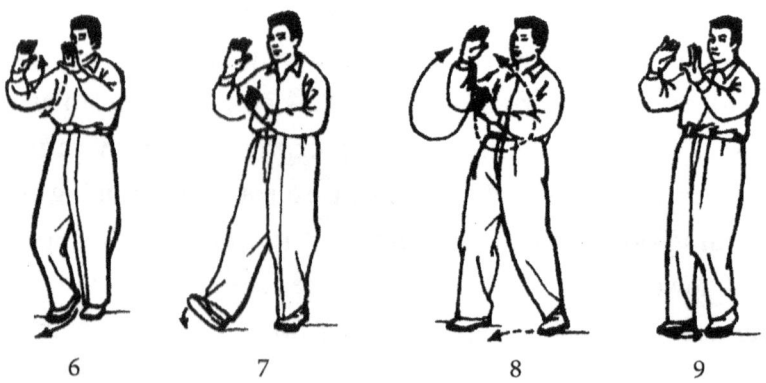

| 6 | 7 | 8 | 9 |

Movement 1:
Look to the south. The right foot moves slightly to the right with the right toe touching the ground. Use the left heel as the axle.

The left toe and the body turn together. The two legs are still left substantial and right insubstantial. Face south. (Figure 6)

Key points: Use intention to change direction. Keep the Body Principles intact.

Movement 2:
Look to the southwest. The body turns slightly to the right. With the turn, the right leg lifts to take a step to the southwest. The toe is up, and the heel is touching the ground. The legs are still left substantial and right insubstantial. At the same time, the right hand, in the vertical palm position, moves downward and then upward in a curve to the height of the shoulder. The left vertical palm moves downward in a curve to the height of the chest. The right arm draws a slightly larger circle than the left hand and is outside and above. The left hand is inside and below. Face southwest. (Figure 7)

Key points: When the two arms move in a curve, the shoulder needs to relax, and the elbows need to sink and feel an attraction to the chest. There needs to be the intention and the sensation of gathering and leading the opponent's incoming force, as well as a feeling of being round and lively. The body needs the energy of folding. The upper and lower body need to coordinate harmoniously.

Movements 3 and 4 are similar to Left Lan Zha Yi, form number 2, Movements 3 and 4. The key points are the same, except the left and right movements are toward different directions and at different angles. (Figures 8, 9)

4. Single Whip (Figures 10-12)

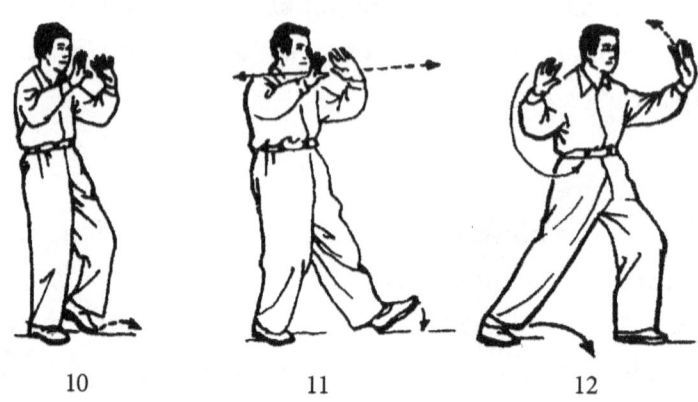

10   11   12

5. Lift Hand (Figure 13)

These two forms together make a sequence. Please notice that Movements 1, 2 and 3 are (initiate, engage and express) Single Whip. Movement 4 (converge) is Lift Hand.

Movement 1:

The left foot moves slightly to the left with the left toe touching the ground. Using the right heel as the axle, the right toe and the body turn 90 degrees to the left together. The eyes look toward the southeast. The legs still are right substantial and left insubstantial. Face southeast. (Figure 10)

Key points: While turning, the body is stable, and the two arms should not move. The left chest contains the intention of being more spacious. Be sure the Body Principles like Relax Shoulder and Sink Elbow are maintained.

Movement 2:

The arms do not move. The left leg takes a step to the east. The toe points up with the heel landing on the ground. The two legs are still right substantial and left insubstantial. (Figure 11)

Key points: When taking a step to the left, Spirit is focused on the right leg. The Body Principles are intact.

Movement 3:
The right heel pushes and the left leg shifts forward forming a curve. The left foot lands flat on the ground, and the body moves forward at the same time. The legs are still right substantial and left insubstantial. Simultaneously, the two vertical palms separate to the left and right, with the left hand at shoulder height and the right hand lower. Face east and slightly to the south. (Figure 12)

Key points: Just before the right heel pushes, begin to gather energy. The tiger mouths (the area between the thumb and first finger), the back of the hands and both shoulders, need to feel that they are connected, with a sensation of being attracted to each other. The Jin, gathered in the two legs, needs to be coupled harmoniously with the two arms. While the right heel pushes, the body needs to stay centered, using the movement of the legs to direct the movement of the arms. At the same time, it is necessary to be attentive to relaxing the shoulder and sinking the elbow.

5. Lift Hand (Figure 13)

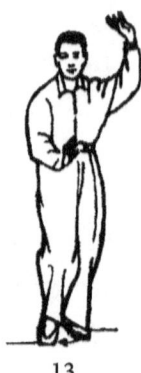

13

Movement 4:

Look to the south. Using the left heel as the axle, the left toe turns slightly to the southeast and the foot lands flat. Immediately switch the left leg to substantial and the right leg to insubstantial. The right leg rises and gathers close to the left leg with the right toe touching the ground. At the same time, the body turns slightly to the right to face south. Both arms move as the body turns, with the right vertical palm moving downward in a curvilinear motion to the hip, then continuing toward the left and stopping in front of the right abdominal area with the fingers pointing forward. The left hand lifts above the forehead with the palm facing upward. (Figure 13)

Key points: When the left hand rises, the left shoulder should not move up. Instead, it should relax and sink down. The palm has the intention of lifting. Simultaneously, the right hand moves downward and outward in a curve. It needs to have rising intention without disconnecting or dispersing the energy. During the entire process the upper and lower body need to harmonize, and attention must be paid to the Body Principles.

6. White Swan Spreads Wings (Figures 14-17)

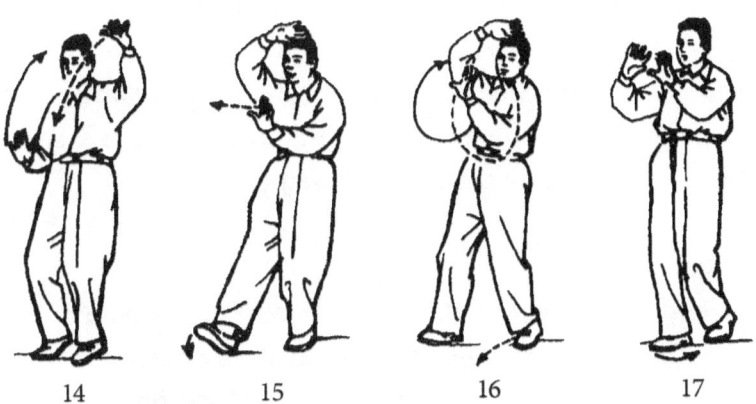

14   15   16   17

Movement 1:

Using the left heel as the axle, turn the left toe toward the south and place it flat on the ground. At the same time, the body turns slightly to the right. The legs are still left substantial and right insubstantial. Face south. (Figure 14)

Key points: The body does not have any significant movement, and the two arms do not move. Maintain the Body Principles.

Movement 2:

Look to the southwest. The right leg steps to the southwest. The toe points up with the heel landing first. The two legs are still left substantial and right insubstantial. At the same time, the right hand rises from the chest to above the eyes with the palm in a horizontal position and the edge of the palm facing forward. The left hand changes to a vertical palm as it moves downward past the right hand and stops in front of the chest. (Figure 15)

Key points: When the right arm is moving up, the right side of the chest should have the intention of sinking downward. There should also be the intention and the sensation of lifting the right leg and stepping forward. After the completion of the movement, the hands form a T shape with the sensation of being connected.

Movement 3:
The left foot pushes and the right leg shifts forward forming a curve. The right foot lands flat and the body moves forward. The legs are still left substantial and right insubstantial. The left vertical palm pushes forward in a southwest direction at chest height. In the meantime, the right hand turns up to a horizontal position. Face southwest. (Figure 16)

Key points: When the left hand pushes forward, the right hand should not lose energy. As the right hand rises, the shoulder needs to relax down and the elbow needs to sink. The body remains centered, and the abdomen is relaxed.

Movement 4:
Still looking to the southwest. The right hand extends forward slightly, the right elbow drops down, and both arms move downward together with vertical palms. On reaching the level of the hips, the arms separate and move left and right and then rise upward in a curve. The arms converge in front of the chest with the fingertips at the height of the shoulder, as if pushing a ball. When the arms start to move upward, the legs change to right substantial and left insubstantial. The left leg moves forward to the right leg, with the toe landing next to the right heel. Face southwest. (Figure 17)

Key points: In the beginning, the rate of the left hand falling is slower than that of the right hand, but when the hands even up, they move together. Other reminders: Please review Movement number 4 of the 2nd form (left Lan Zha Yi) for key points.

7. Brush Knee Twist Step (Figures 18-21)

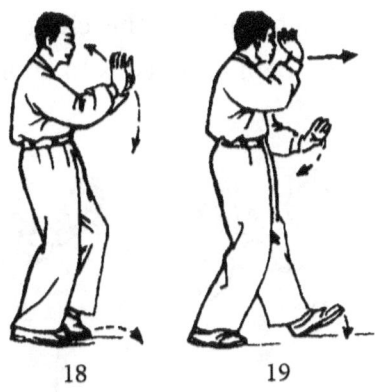

18   19

Movement 1:
The left foot moves to behind the right foot, with the toe touching the ground. Together, using the left heel as the axle, the body and the right toe turn 135 degrees to the left. The legs are right substantial and left insubstantial. (Figure 18)

Key points: When turning, the eyes initiate the action. The body and the right toe need to move together in lockstep.

Movement 2:
Look to the northeast. The body turns slightly to the left. The left leg starts to step to the northeast with the toe pointing up. The heel lands first. The legs are still right substantial

and left insubstantial. At the same time, the left vertical palm moves from the left side of the chest, dropping to the left abdominal area. The right vertical palm moves from the right side of the chest and rises to the right side of the face. Face northeast. (Figure 19)

Key points: The up and down motion of the two arms should have the intention of separating the opponent from his strength. The falling left hand needs to have the intention of connection with the left chest. When the right hand is moving up, the right side of the chest should have the intention of sinking down and needs to coordinate with the left foot stepping.

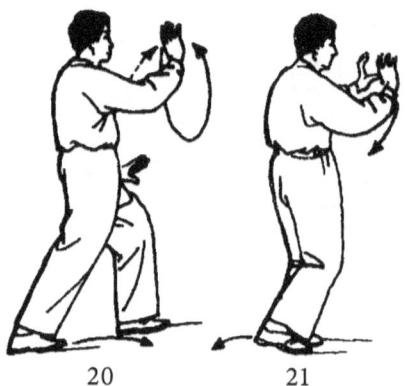

20   21

Movement 3:

The right heel pushes, and the left leg shifts forward forming a curve. The left foot lands flat, and the body moves forward. The legs are still right substantial and left insubstantial. At the same time, the left hand moves downward, brushes above the left knee and stops just outside of the left leg, with the palm facing downward, and the fingers pointing forward. The right vertical palm slowly pushes forward and northeast at the height of the mouth. Face northeast. (Figure 20)

Key points: When the left hand drops toward the knee, it needs to be controlled by the left chest, which is directing the movement of the left hand. At the same time, the right hand and the right shoulder should feel connected and attracted to each other, with the energy of leading and gathering. When the right hand pushes forward, the palm should have the intention of sinking. When the left hand is moving to the outside of the left leg, it should have the intention of supporting the right hand pushing forward. At this time the body should not turn.

Movement 4:
Continue to look to the northeast. The right vertical palm drops to the front of the right hip with the fingers of both hands pointing forward. The hands then separate to the right and left as they lift upward in a curve. The vertical palms converge in front of the chest as if ready to push a ball. When the arms are rising, the two legs change to left substantial and right insubstantial. The right leg moves up next to the left foot with the right toe touching the ground. Face northeast. (Figure 21)

Key points: When the left hand is dropping, the fingers should have a rising intention. At the same time, the right shoulder needs to have the intention of pulling the arm. During this time the body energy should stay vibrant, without dispersing. Keep the sensation of suspension. While stepping up, the body needs to have the intention of gathering and converging.

8. Play the Guitar (Figure 22)

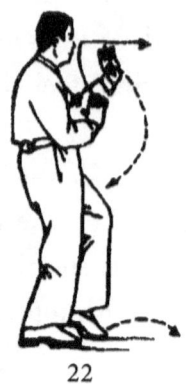

22

9. Brush Knee Twist Step (Figures 23-26)

These two forms together form a sequence. Movement 1 is Play the Guitar. Movements 2, 3 and 4 are Brush Knee Twist Step.

Movement 1:
The right foot steps back and lands flat, with the toe pointing to the east. The legs change to right substantial and left insubstantial. The left foot gathers back to the left front side of the right foot with the toe touching the ground. At the same time, the two vertical palms retreat and gather as the body shifts backward. The left hand is at shoulder height and the right hand drops to the front of the right side of the abdomen. Face northeast. (Figure 22)

Key points: When stepping back with the right foot, the buttocks must not move back. Spirit focuses on the upper right thigh. After the right foot lands flat, and the right upper thigh has strength, one can lift the left leg and move it back. At the same time, the forward intention should still be there.

The chest needs to relax and sink down, with the intention of making a curve from up to down. Use this intention to lead and coordinate the movement of the arms. The space between the arms and the chest needs to feel round and lively. The buttocks should have the intention of going forward to gather the two arms in toward the body. Simultaneously, relax the abdomen and open the space around the waist wide, with a feeling of getting bigger.

Movement 2:
Continue to look in the same direction. The left leg steps forward with the toes pointing up and the heel landing first. The legs are still right substantial and left insubstantial. At the same time, the left vertical palm moves from the front of the left chest and drops to the front of the left abdomen. The right vertical palm moves from the front of the right chest and rises to the right side of the face (like Figure 19). Afterward, the right heel pushes forward, the left leg shifts forward with a curve, and the left foot lands flat as the body moves forward. The two legs are still right substantial and left insubstantial. Simultaneously, the left hand drops down, brushes over the top of the left knee and stops at the side of the left leg with the palm facing down and the fingers pointing forward. The right vertical palm extends slowly forward toward the northeast at the height of the mouth. Face northeast. (Figure 23)

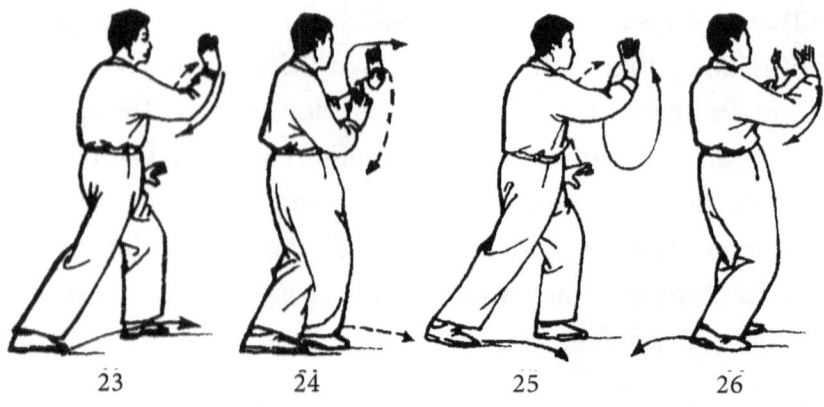

23   24   25   26

The legs change to left substantial and right insubstantial. Lift the right leg and cross over the left foot, with the right foot landing flat in front of the left foot. The legs change to right substantial and left insubstantial. Next, the left vertical palm rises to shoulder height, and the right vertical palm drops lower to the front of the chest. Face northeast. (Figure 24)

Key points: The key points for Figure 23 are the same as those of the 7th form (Brush Knee Twist Step), Movements 2 and 3.

In the crossover in Figure 24, the arms and the chest should feel attracted and connected. At the same time, the body needs to feel like it is gathering and converging. Be attentive to the transformation of insubstantial to substantial during the steps.

The explanation of Movements 2 and 3 in this form Figure 23 are the same, and the key points are the same. (Figure 25)

Movement 4 and the 7th form (Brush Knee Twist Step) Movement 4 Figure 21 are the same, and the key points are the same. (Figure 26)

10. Play the Guitar (Figure 27)

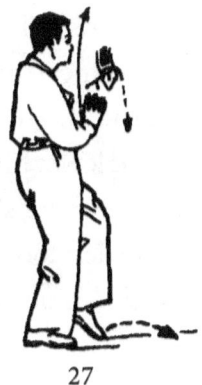

27

11: Step Forward, Parry, Repulse and Punch
(Figure 28-30.1 and Figure 30.2)

These two forms together form a sequence. Movement 1 is Play the Guitar. Movements 2, 3 and 4 are Step Forward, Parry, Repulse and Punch.

Movement 1:
The description of Movement 1 is the same as for the 8th form, Play the Guitar. The key points are the same. (Figure 27)

Movement 2:
(Left Step Forward): The direction stays the same. The right leg steps forward with the toe pointing up. The heel lands first. The right hand turns from vertical palm to thumbs up with the other four fingers pointing forward. All five fingers extend comfortably, with the palm facing left. Next, the right hand extends upward and stops in front of the right forehead. Simultaneously, the left vertical palm drops down in front of the left abdomen.

Next, the right foot pushes, the left leg shifts forward to form a curve, and the left foot lands flat with the body moving forward. The legs are still right substantial and left insubstantial. At the same time, both arms extend gently forward. Face northeast. (Figure 28)

Key points: The upper and lower limbs need to coordinate. When the right arm is rising, there should be the intention and the feeling of leading the left foot as it steps forward. Do not let the energy disperse. Focus on one direction. The body should not lean to any side.

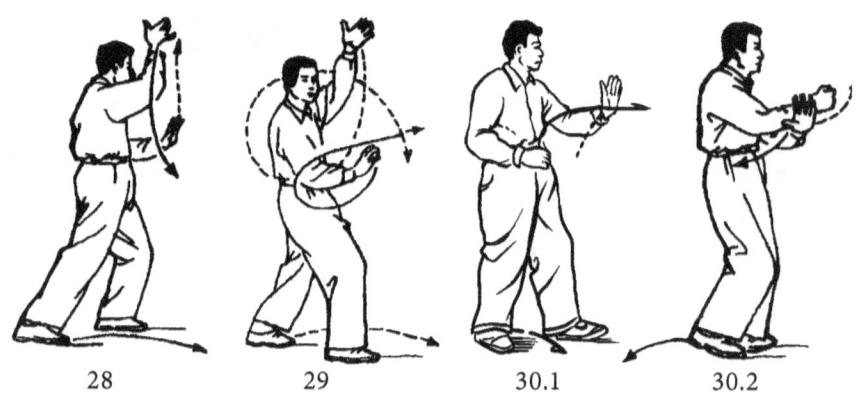

| 28 | 29 | 30.1 | 30.2 |

Movement 3:

(Right Step Forward): Using the left heel as the axle, the left toe turns right, to the east, and lands flat facing southeast. The body turns slightly to the right. After the legs change to left substantial and right insubstantial, lift the right leg close to the left leg and then step forward toward the southeast with the heel landing first. The left thumb turns and points upward with the four fingers pointing forward. The fingers extend comfortably, and the palm faces right. Extend the palm to the upper left and stop in front of the left forehead.

The right vertical palm drops down in front of the right side of the abdomen. Next, the left foot pushes and shifts the left leg forward, forming a curve. The left foot lands flat as the body moves forward. The legs are still left substantial and right insubstantial. Simultaneously, both arms extend gently forward. Face southeast. (Figure 29)

Key points: Use intention to lead the changes of direction. Spirit focuses on the right leg after completing the transformation of insubstantial to substantial. Only then can the right leg step forward. Other key points are the same as for Movement 2 of this form, only the direction and angle are different. Left and right are in reverse.

Movement 4:
(Parry, Repulse and Punch): Look to the east. The left vertical palm drops from in front of the face, curving to the left. At the front of the hip, the hand moves straight to the left and then circles back to the east in a big circle. From the front of the chest, it drops to the left front of the abdomen, still in the vertical palm position. Next, the two legs change to right substantial and left insubstantial. The left leg moves up to near the right leg and then steps to the east with the heel landing first. At the same time, the right arm drops gently to the right hip and the hand forms a vertical fist. (Figure 30.1)

Next, the left leg bends forward, the left foot lands flat, and the body moves forward. The legs then change to left substantial right insubstantial. The right leg moves forward next to the left leg with the toe touching the ground. Next, the left vertical palm pulls slightly inward while the right fist strikes forward and passes over the top of the left hand at the height of the heart, with the fist vertical. Face east. (Figure 30.2)

117

Key points: When the left hand is drawing a curve, the left chest should feel light, with energy sinking down to direct the movement of the left arm. The left shoulder should have the sensation of pulling and connection with the left hand. The drawing of the curve needs to proceed seamlessly. When the left hand is drawing the curve upwards, there needs to be the intention of lifting and leading the left leg stepping forward. When striking with the right fist, the right elbow should have the intention of sinking, and the right arm should have the intention of lifting and leading the right leg forward. At the same time, one needs to pay attention to the transformation of the insubstantial and the substantial and the body folding requirement.

12. Withdraw and Push (Figures 31-34)

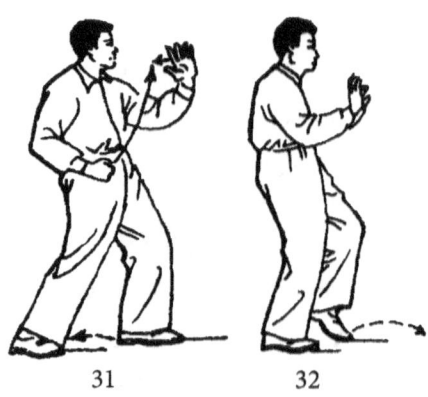

31   32

Movement 1:

The direction stays the same. The left leg does not move, the right leg and right fist move back together, the right leg takes a step backward and to the side behind the left heel, and the toe points to the southeast and lands flat. The legs are still left substantial and right insubstantial. The right vertical fist stops at the side of the right hip. Simultaneously, the left vertical palm moves upward to the left front of the chest. (Figure 31)

Key points: While stepping back, maintain the stability of the body. The body does not shift back. The two arms should be attentive to sinking the elbow.

Movement 2:

Face the same direction. The right fist changes to the vertical palm position and moves upward to the right front of the chest at the same height as the left hand. The legs transform to right substantial and left insubstantial. The body follows the action and moves backward. The left leg gathers back with the left toe touching the ground. While the body is moving back, gather both arms inward to the front of the chest. (Figure 32)

Key points: Before the body moves back, the buttocks need to gather forward slightly. At the same time the tailbone needs to stand up to be able to transform Jin. While the body is moving back, it needs to stay centered. The space between the arms and the chest needs to feel round and lively.

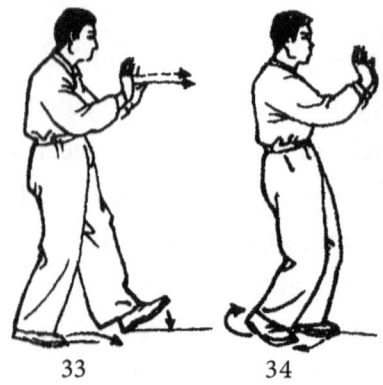

33   34

Movement 3:

Face the same direction. The left leg steps forward with the toe pointing up. The heel lands first. The two legs are still right substantial and left insubstantial. (Figure 33)

Key points: Before stepping, be attentive to Spirit. The focus continues to be on the right leg, and stepping should feel like stepping on thin ice.

Movement 4:

The left leg bends slightly, and the left foot lands flat. Next, the two legs transform to left substantial and right insubstantial. The right leg moves forward with the toe touching down next to the left foot. While the right leg is moving up, both vertical palms extend gently forward at the height of the chest. Face east. (Figure 34)

Key points: When the left leg is bending, both arms and both shoulders should feel connected and like they are pulling each other, with the feeling of leading and gathering. While the two hands are pushing forward, they need to have the intention of sinking. Relax the shoulder and sink the elbow. The body should not lean forward or backward.

13. Carry Tiger, Push Mountain (Figures 35-38)

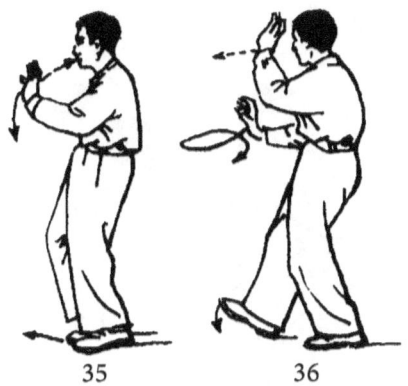

35   36

Movement 1:

The right leg steps back to behind the left foot with the toe touching the ground. Using the left heel as the axle, the left toe and body move together and turn around to the right 180 degrees. Face west. The legs are still left substantial and right insubstantial. (Figure 35)

Key points: When the body turns around to the right, it needs to be stable and follow Tai Ji Quan's methods of energy transformation.

Movement 2:

Look to the northwest. The body turns slightly to the right, and the hands and feet shift with it. The left leg steps to the northwest, and the toe points up with the heel landing first. The legs are still left substantial and right insubstantial. The right vertical palm drops down to the front of the right abdomen while the left vertical palm rises to the right side of the face. Face northwest. (Figure 36)

Key points: The movement of the two arms needs to include the intention of leading and transforming. At the same time the whole body needs to coordinate to maintain the Body Principles.

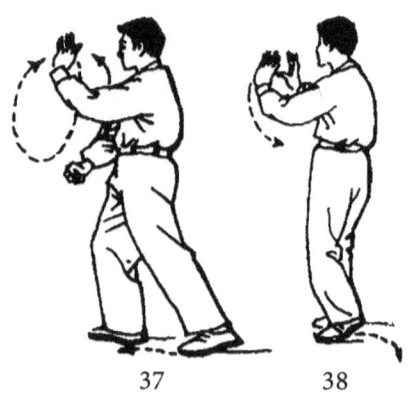

37   38

Movement 3:

Look to the northwest. The right vertical palm starts from in front of the abdomen and moves left and then forward. Next, it moves to the right in a circular motion to the right side of the abdomen and changes to a fist, with the inside of the fist facing the chest. The right arm forms the shape of carrying a tiger. Next, the left foot pushes, and the right leg shifts forward forming a curve. The right foot lands flat, and the body shifts forward. At the same time, the left vertical palm extends gently forward toward the northwest. The left hand is at the height of the mouth, and the right arm feels that it is expanding outward. The two legs are still left substantial and right insubstantial. Face northwest. (Figure 37)

Key points: The curving movement of the right arm is directed by the right side of the chest and needs to include the intention of meeting and receiving the opponent's incoming force, using the energy of engage and gathering. When the right foot pushes against the ground, the right arm carrying the tiger needs to feel full, and the left hand needs to have the sensation of sinking. The whole body needs to coordinate.

Movement 4:
The direction is the same. The right fist turns so that the palm faces down, drops to the side of the right hip and then changes to the vertical palm position. At the same time, the left hand, with the palm vertical, drops to the side of the left hip. Next, the two arms separate to the left and right sides and move upward in a curve. Both palms meet in front of the chest in a position like pushing a ball. The two hands are at shoulder height. When the arms start to draw an upward curve, the legs transform to right substantial and left insubstantial. Next, the left foot follows up to the side of the right heel with the toe touching the ground. Face northwest. (Figure 38)

Key points: In the beginning the left hand falls slightly faster than the right hand. Once the hands are even, the hands move together smoothly. At the same time both shoulders should have the intention of attracting and pulling the arms. Before stepping up, the Jin needs to transform with the tailbone standing. While stepping, the whole body needs to have the intention of gathering and converging combined with the intention of expansion within convergence.

14. Play the Guitar (Figure 39)

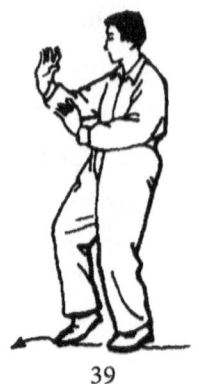

39

15. Right Lan Zha Yi (Figure 40-42)

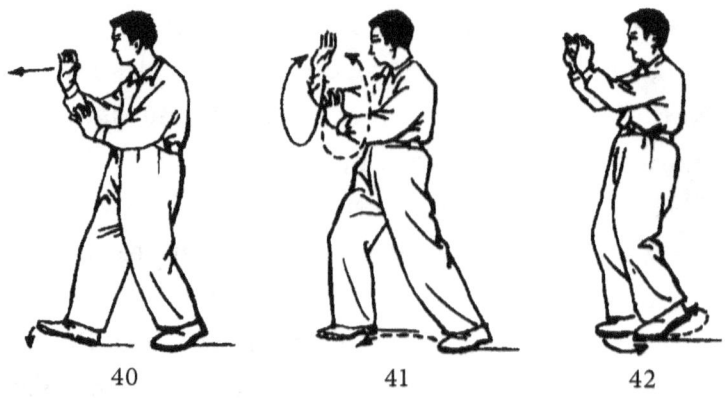

40   41   42

These two forms together form a sequence. Movement 1 is Play the Guitar. Movements 2, 3 and 4 are Right Lan Zha Yi.

Movement 1:
Look to the west. The left leg steps back and lands flat. The toe points to the southwest. The legs are left substantial and right insubstantial. The right foot moves in front of the left foot with the toe touching the ground. As the body turns left and

the foot moves back, both vertical palms gather in front of the chest with the right hand at shoulder height and the left hand dropping to the left side of the abdomen. Face west. (Figure 39)

Key points: When the body turns left, one needs to maintain the Body Principles.

The other key points are the same as the 8th form, Play the Guitar, except that the direction and angle of the movements are reversed.

Movement 2:
The right leg steps forward, and the toe points up with the heel landing first. The legs are still left substantial and right insubstantial. (Figure 40)

Key points: Maintain the Body Principles. Although the hand does not move, nevertheless, the intention of the hands and the movement of the right leg are connected.

Movements 3 and 4 are similar to the 3rd form Right Lan Zha Yi Movements 3 and 4, but in a different direction. This form faces west. The key points are the same as the 3rd form Movements 3 and 4. (Figures 41, 42)

16. Single Whip (Figures 43-45)

17. Lift Hand (Figure 46)

The two forms together form a sequence. Movement 1, 2 and 3 are Single Whip. Movement 4 is Lift Hand.

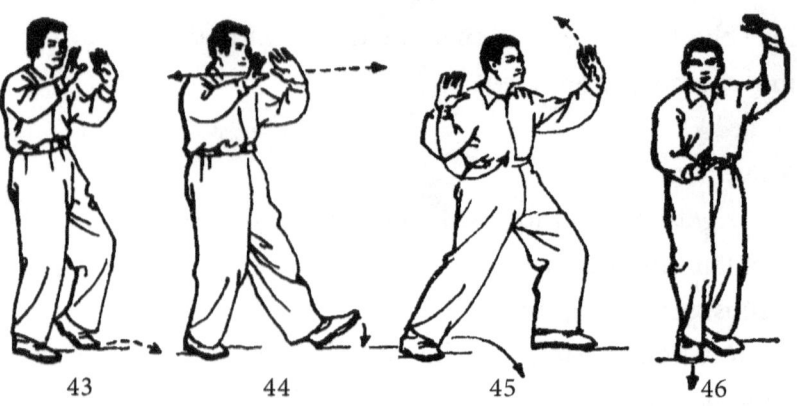

43   44   45   46

Movement 1:

The left foot rises and moves back to the left side of the right foot, with the toe touching the ground. Next, using the right heel as the axle, the right toe and body turn together to the left 135 degrees. (Figure 43) The legs are still right substantial and left insubstantial. Face east and slightly to the south.

Key points: The points are similar to the 4th form Single Whip, only the turn is greater than 90 degrees.

Movements 2 and 3 are similar to the 4th form Single Whip Movement 2 and 3. The key points are the same. (Figures 44, 45)

Movement 4 is the same as the 5th form Lift Hand. The key points are the same. (Figure 46)

18. Fist Under Elbow (Figures 47-50)

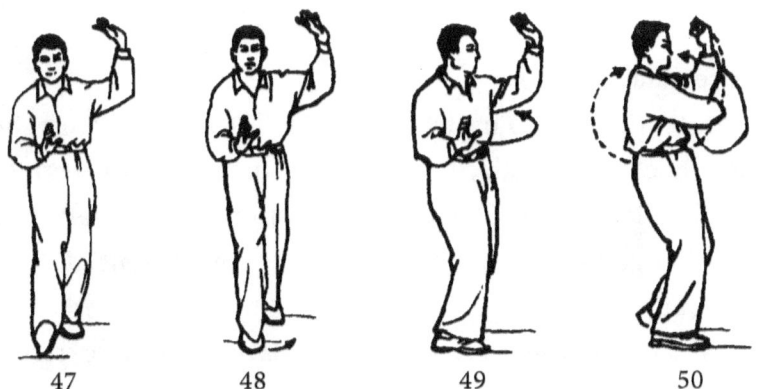

47   48   49   50

Movement 1:

The right leg steps forward with the toe up. The heel lands first. The legs are left substantial and right insubstantial. At the same time, the right vertical palm rises to the front of the chest. Face south. (Figure 47)

Key points: The right leg steps out and is directed and supported by the left leg, while at the same time the right hand and right leg coordinate together. The lifting energy of the left hand should not be loose or absent. Maintain the Body Principles.

Movement 2:

The left heel pushes and the right leg shifts forward forming a curve. The right foot lands flat and the body shifts forward with the right vertical palm pushing forward gently at chest height. Face south. (Figure 48)

Key points: The left hand has the intention of lifting. Be attentive to relaxing the shoulder and sinking the elbow. The right hand that pushes forward should have the intention of sinking. The upper and lower body need to coordinate. The body should not lean forward or backward.

Movement 3:
Look to the east. The left leg does not move. Using the right heel as the axle, the right toe turns left 90 degrees and then lands flat. The waist turns slightly to the left. The legs change to right substantial and left insubstantial. Face east. (Figure 49)

Key point: The body should not have excessive external turning.

Movement 4:
Both vertical palms convert to fists, and the body turns left to the east. While the right fist moves to the left with the back of the fist under the left elbow, the left front of the hip straightens. The left fist is at the same height as the top of the head and faces inward. By turning the body, the left foot comes next to the right heel, with the toe touching the ground. The legs are still right substantial and left insubstantial. Face east. (Figure 50)

Key points: Both sides of the chest need to direct the motion of the arms. Simultaneously, the chest and the upper arm need to feel expanded, round and lively. When the left foot moves close to the right foot, the right waist eye needs to lift the left waist eye. The abdomen is relaxed.

19. Left Repulse Monkey (Figures 51-54)

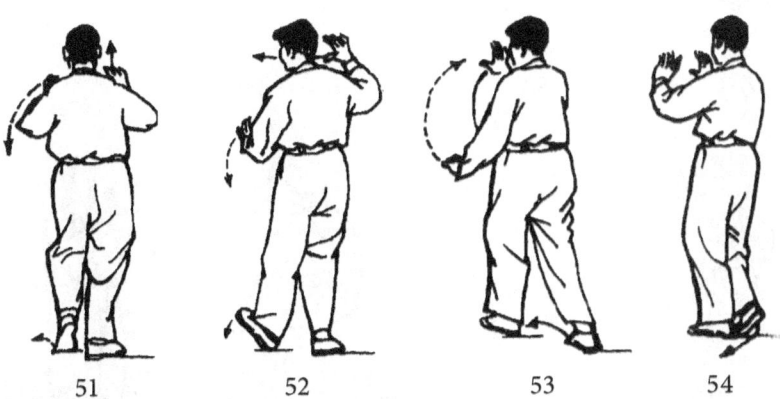

51   52   53   54

Movement 1:

The left foot moves left to behind the right heel with the toe touching the ground. Then, using the right heel as the axle, the left toe and body turn together to the left 90 degrees. At the same time, both hands change from fists to vertical palms, first drawing a curve downward and then separating to the left and right and moving up to and meet in front of the chest at shoulder height as if they were pushing a ball. The two legs are still right substantial and left insubstantial. Face north. (Figure 51)

Key points: When the arms are drawing a curve, they need to coordinate with the body's left turn. The left curve should be slightly larger between the chest and the upper arms and should feel round and lively and maintain the Body Principles.

Movements 2, 3 and 4 are the same as the 7th form Brush Knee Twist Step Movements 2, 3 and 4. The key points are the same, only the direction and angle are different. The direction of the movement is northwest. Face northwest. (Figures 52 – 54)

20. Right Repulse Monkey (Figures 55-58)

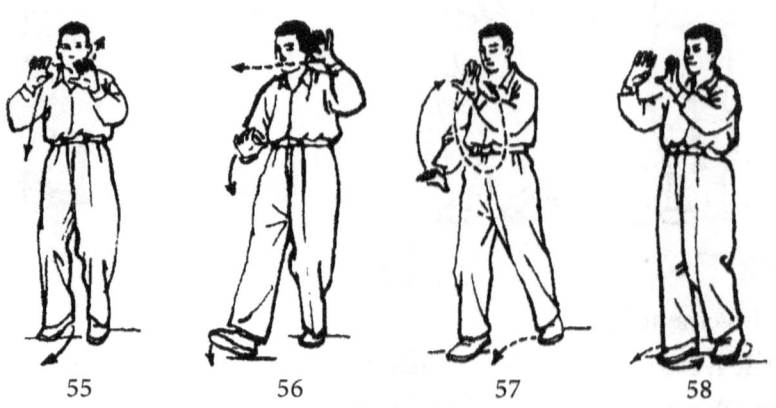

| 55 | 56 | 57 | 58 |

Movement 1:
Lift the right toe and move it to the left side of the left heel with the toe touching the ground. Next, using the left heel as the axle, the left toe and the body turn together 225 degrees to the right. The legs are still left substantial and right insubstantial. Face south. (Figure 55)

Key points: While turning, the right side of the chest should have the intention of being more spacious, and the body should maintain stability.

Movement 2:
Look to the southwest. The body turns slightly to the right, and the hands and feet start to move with the turn. The right leg steps to the southwest. The heel lands first with the toe pointing upward. The legs are still left substantial and right insubstantial. At the same time, the

right vertical palm falls to the right side of the abdomen, and the left vertical palm moves to the left side of the face. Face southwest. (Figure 56)

Key points: The key points are the same as the 7th form Brush Knee Twist Step Movements 2, only with the direction and the angle different. The left and right movements are opposite.

Movement 3:

Keep the same direction. The left heel pushes, and the right leg shifts forward forming a curve. The right foot lands flat, with the body moving forward. The right hand moves downward, brushes over the right knee and stops to the outside of the right leg with the palm facing down, and the fingers pointing forward. The left vertical palm faces forward (southwest) and gently pushes forward at the height of the mouth. (Figure 57)

Key points: The key points are the same as for the 7th form (Brush Knee Twist Step) Movement 3, with the directions and angle different, and the left and right movements reversed.

Movement 4:

The left vertical palm drops down to the side of the left hip at the same height as the right hand. Next, the two hands separate to the left and right, drawing a curve upwards with the vertical palms meeting in front of chest at shoulder height as if pushing a ball. When the hands begin to move upward, the legs change to right substantial and left insubstantial. Then the left leg moves up next to the right leg with the toe touching the ground. Face southwest. (Figure 58)

Key points: The key points are the same as for the 7th form (Brush Knee Twist Step) movements, except that the direction and angle are different and the left and right movements are reversed.

21. Left Repulse Monkey (Figures 59-62)

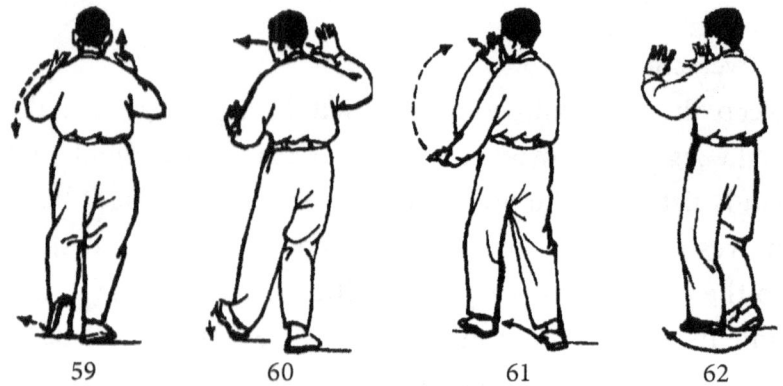

| 59 | 60 | 61 | 62 |

Movement 1:
Lift the left foot and move it to the right side of the right heel with the toe touching the ground. Next, using the right heel as the axle, the right toe and the body turn 225 degrees together to the back. The legs are still right substantial and left insubstantial. Face north. (Figure 59)

Key points: When turning, the left side of the chest should have the intention of spaciousness. The body needs to maintain stability.

Movements 2, 3 and 4 are the same as the for the 7th form (Brush Knee Twist Step) Movements 2, 3 and 4. Only the direction and angle are different. This form moves to the northwest and faces northwest. The key points are the same. (Figure 60 – 62)

22. Right Repulse Monkey (Figures 63-66)

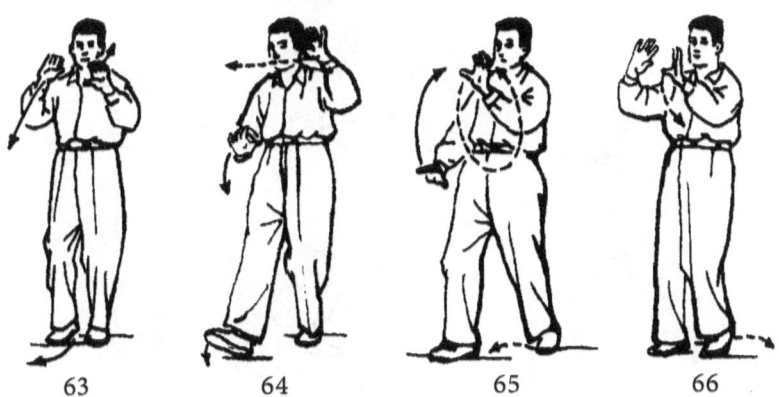

63   64   65   66

Movements 1, 2, 3 and 4:

The key points are the same as for the 20th form (Right Repulse Monkey). (Figures 63 – 66)

23. Play the Guitar (Figure 67)

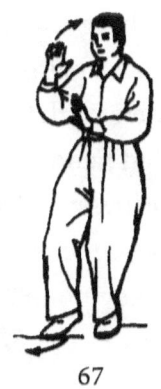

67

24. White Swan Spreads Wings (Figure 68-70)

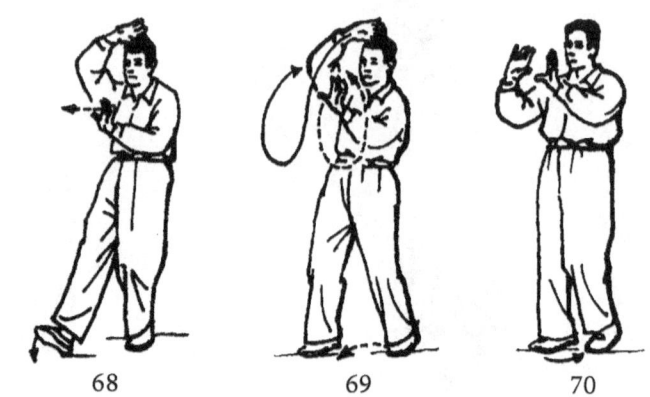

68   69   70

These two forms form a sequence. Movement 1 is Play the Guitar, Movements 2, 3 and 4 are White Swan Spreads Wings.

Movement 1:

The left leg steps back and lands flat with the toe pointing south. Next, the two legs change to left substantial and right insubstantial. The right foot gathers to the right side of the left foot with the toe touching the ground. While the right foot is moving, both vertical palms move back toward the body. The right hand gathers back to the front of the chest at shoulder height, and the left hand drops down to the left side of the abdomen. Face southwest. (Figure 67)

Key points: This is the same movement as the 8th form (Play the Guitar) and the key points are the same. Only the left and right movements are opposite, with the direction and angles different.

Movement 2:

Keep the same direction. The right leg steps forward, the heel touches the ground with the toe pointing up. The legs are still left substantial and right insubstantial. When the right vertical palm rises diagonally up to the forehead and changes to the palm facing forward, the left vertical palm moves to the front of the chest. (Figure 68)

Key points: When the right hand is lifting, the right side of the chest needs to have a sinking sensation along with the intention of leading and lifting the right leg while stepping forward. The left chest needs to direct the left arm to move up. After completing the movement, the two hands form a T shape and need to feel connected. Maintain the Body Principles.

Movements 3 and 4 are the same as the 6th form (White Swan Spreads Wings) Movement 3 and 4. The key points are similar.

25. Brush Knee Twist Step (Figures 71-74)

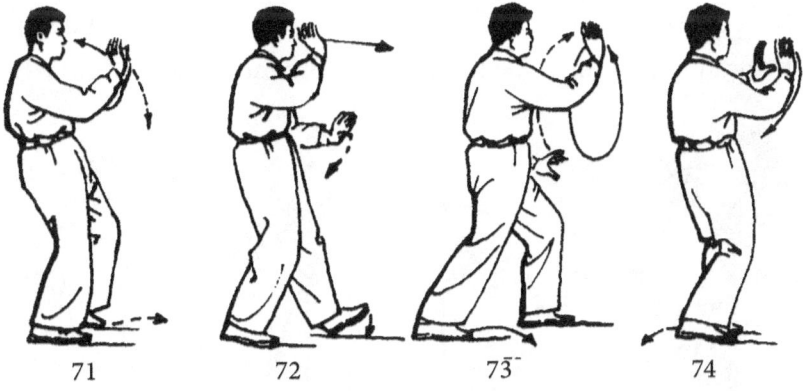

71   72   73   74

Movements 1, 2, 3 and 4:
The key points are the same as the 7th form Brush Knee Twist Step. (Figures 71 – 74)

26. Play the Guitar (Figure 75)

27. Press Down (Figure 76)

28. Green Dragon Rises Out of Water
(Figures 77.1, 77.2)

29. Turn Around (Figures 78.1, 78.2)

These four forms complete a sequence with Movement 1 (Play the Guitar), Movement 2 (Press Down), Movement 3 (Green Dragon Rises Out of Water) and Movement 4 (Turn Around).

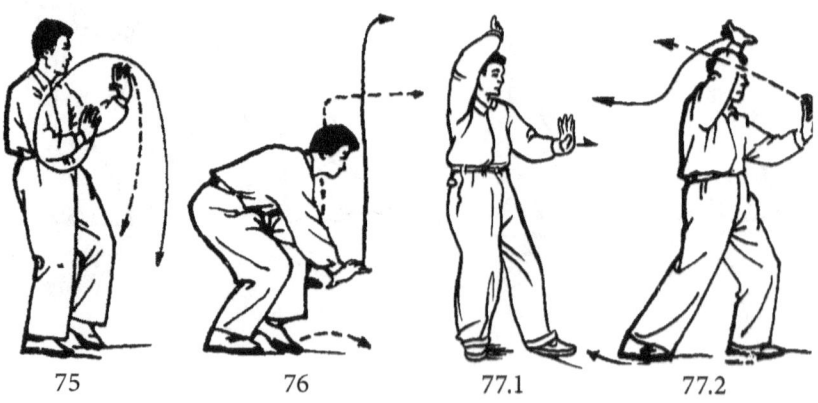

75   76   77.1   77.2

Movement 1:

The right leg steps back and lands flat with the toe pointing to the southeast. Look east. The legs change to right substantial and left insubstantial. Next, the left foot gathers to the front of the left side of the right foot with the toe pointing to the ground. At the same time, the two vertical palms, following the slight turn of the body to the right, gather to the front of the chest with the left hand at shoulder height. The right hand drops to the right front of the abdomen. Face east. (Figure 75)

Key points: The key points are the same as the 8th form (Play the Guitar) except the direction is different. This form faces east.

Movement 2:

The right palm moves to the side and turns to face up with the fingers pointing to the left. It first moves to the right and up, and then moves to the left drawing a curve to the front of the forehead. The palm slowly turns downwards with the fingers still pointing to the left. Simultaneously, the left hand draws a curve starting in front of the chest down to the side of the left hip, with the palm turning and facing down. Together the two hands press down. The upper body leans forward and moves downward while bending the knees to lower the body. The left fingers point forward and move to the left side of the left calf, with the right fingers pointing to the left and moving in front of the two knees. The legs are still right substantial and left insubstantial. Face east. (Figure 76)

Key points: the movement of the arms should include the intention of following the opponent's incoming force and gathering to the front of the chest. Continue to follow the energy while bending down with the legs. The body leans forward and downward but does not tip forward. Spirit is focused on the upper thigh of the right leg. The chest and back need to relax and sink. Look forward and not straight down to the ground.

Movement 3:

The direction is the same. Lift the body up. At the same time, the right forearm lifts diagonally to above the forehead with the palm facing upward and forward, and the fingers pointing to the left. The left hand moves upward with a vertical palm to the front of the chest. The left leg steps out forward. The heel lands with the toe pointing upwards. (Figure 77.1)

Immediately afterward, the right heel pushes, the left leg moves forward forming a curve, the left foot lands flat, and the toe points to the east with the body moving forward. The two legs continue to be right substantial and left insubstantial. At the same time, the left hand slowly pushes forward with the fingertips at the height of the chest. (Figure 77.2)

Key points: While the body is straightening, it needs to maintain all the Body Principles, and the two rising arms must proceed with down intention first. The left hand, which is pushing forward, should have the intention of sinking, while the right hand has the intention of rising. The right shoulder needs to relax and sink down. The upper and lower body need to coordinate.

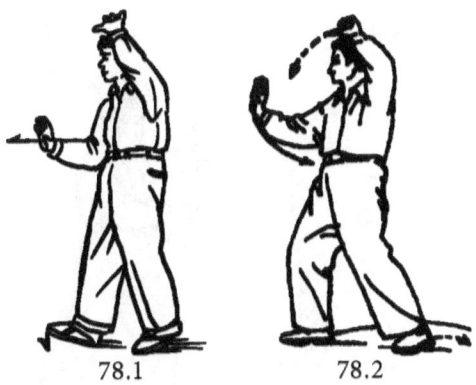

78.1   78.2

Movement 4:

Using the left heel as the axle, the left toe turns right 135 degrees and lands flat. Change the legs to left substantial and right insubstantial. The body turns around to the right and faces west. The right leg lifts and then drops to the front and right side of the left foot with the heel landing first and the toe pointing to the west. Simultaneously, the left hand lifts above the forehead with the palm facing forward and upward. The fingers point to the right. The right vertical palm drops to the front of the chest. (Figure 78.1)

Immediately afterwards, the left heel pushes, and the right leg moves forward forming a curve. The right foot lands flat with the body moving forward. The legs are still left substantial and right insubstantial. At the same time, the right vertical palm pushes forward slowly at chest height. The left hand has similar energy moving forward. Face west. (Figure 78.2)

Key points: When turning, the body needs to be stable. The movement of the two arms needs to coordinate with the turning of the body. After completing the turn, the arm should be at the proper finish position. Pay attention to the folding and energy exchange.

30. Three Changing Backs (Figures 79-82)

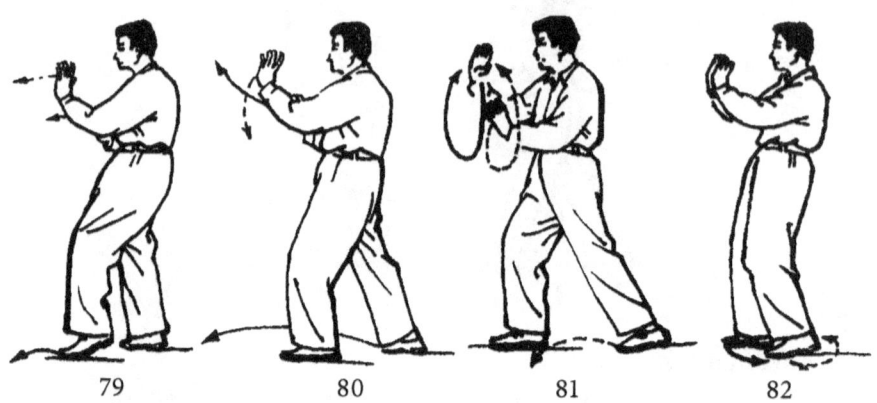

79   80   81   82

Movement 1:

Look to the west. The right leg takes a big step backward and the foot lands flat with the toe pointing to the northwest. The legs change to right substantial and left insubstantial. While the body is moving back, take the left leg back with the toe landing to the left front side of the right foot. Simultaneously, both vertical palms gather backward with the hands at shoulder height and the right hand in front of the chest. Face west. (Figure 79)

Key points: When the body is moving back, pay attention to the transformation of the insubstantial and substantial while maintaining the Body Principles. When the hands gather backward, the chest should have the intention of opening wide. The Qi should stick to the back and sink. The upper and lower body should coordinate and follow each other.

Movement 2:

The direction stays the same. The left leg steps forward with the heel landing on the ground and the toe pointing upward.

Next, the right foot pushes forward, the left leg moves forward forming a curve with the left foot landing flat, and the body moves forward. The legs are still right substantial and left insubstantial. While the right leg is pushing, the two vertical palms push slowly forward with the left hand at shoulder height and the right hand at chest height. (Figure 80)

Key points: The right leg should direct and support the left leg moving forward. When the foot touches the ground, it should feel like stepping on thin ice. The two hands should not move randomly. Other key points are the same as the 2nd form (left Lan Zha Yi) Movement number 3. Only the direction and angle are different.

Movement 3:
The direction stays the same. The left toe turns slightly outward, points to the southwest and lands flat. The legs change to left substantial and right insubstantial. The right leg takes a big step forward with the heel touching the ground and the toe pointing upward. While the right leg is stepping forward, the right vertical palm moves upward in a curve and the left vertical palm moves downward in a curve. Then the left foot pushes forward and the right leg shifts forward forming a curve, with the right foot landing flat and the toe pointing to the west. The body moves forward, and at the same time the two palms push forward slowly, with the right hand at shoulder height and left hand at chest height. (Figure 81)

Key points: While stepping, the upper and lower body need to coordinate and follow each other. As the right hand moves upward, it should have the intention of lifting and leading the right leg forward. Pay attention to the folding and the energy transformation. Other key points are the same as Movement 3 of the 3rd form (Lan Zha Yi).

Movement 4:
Similar to the 3rd form (right Lan Zha Yi) Movement number 4. Only the direction and angle are different. The key points are the same. This form faces west. (Figure 82)

31. Single Whip (Figures 83-85)

32. Down Posture (Figure 86)

A sequence is made from the two forms above. Movement 1, 2 and 3 are Single Whip. Movement 4 is Down Posture.

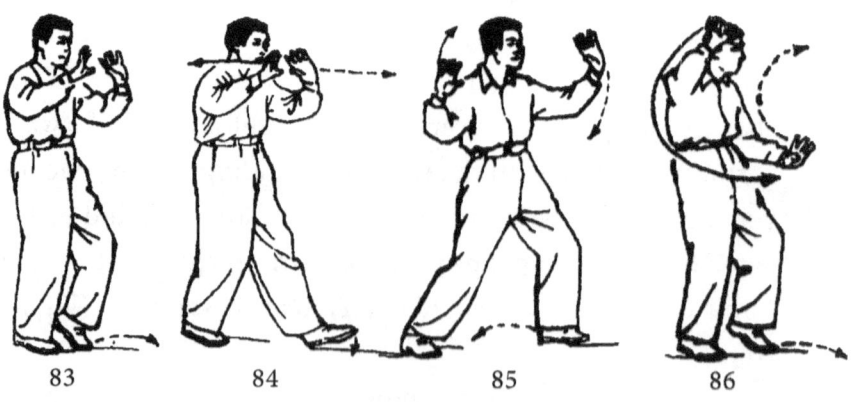

83   84   85   86

Movement 1 and the 16th form (Single Whip) are the same, and the key points are the same. (Figure 83)

Movements 2 and 3 are the same as the 4th form Single Whip Movements 2 and 3. The key points are also the same. (Figures 84, 85)

Movement 4:
Look to the east. The body shifts back slightly and the left foot gathers back to the side of the right foot with the toe pointing to the ground. The legs are right substantial and left insubstantial. At the same time as the left vertical palm drops to the side of the left hip with the arm slightly bent and the right hand rises above the head with the palm facing upward. Face east with the body turned slightly to the south. (Figure 86)

Key points: Before stepping back, focus additional Spirit on the right upper thigh and tailbone. It is necessary to stand with the head and pelvis suspended, the chest relaxed and the back open. Relax the abdomen and maintain the other Body Principles. While stepping back, the body cannot lean forward or backward. The left hand drops and should include the intention of rising. The right hand lifts and should have the intention of holding up the sky.

33. Cloud Hands (Figures 87-90)

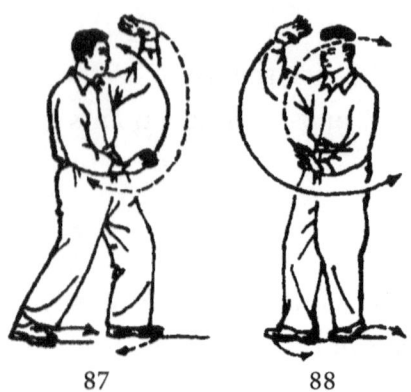

87   88

Movement 1:
Start looking to the southeast. The left leg steps out forward with the heel landing first and the toe pointing up and to the east, in a slight southerly direction. Subsequently, the right heel pushes, the left leg shifts forward forming a curve, and the left foot lands flat with the body moving forward. Simultaneously, the left vertical palm moves in an upward curve from the front of the abdomen. The left forearm moves slowly up diagonally in front of the forehead with the palm facing forward and up. The right vertical palm moves to the right and downward, drawing a half circle to the front of the right abdomen, with the palm facing down. Both hands align in a vertical line. Face southeast. (Figure 87)

Key points: When the left arm is moving up, the left shoulder should not lift. Instead, the left shoulder should relax and sink down. The left chest and left leg should feel connected by a mutual attraction. The movements of both arms need to be round and lively. The upper and lower body need to coordinate.

Movement 2:

Using the left heel as the axle, the left toe turns inward toward the south and lands flat. The legs change to left substantial and right insubstantial. Look to the southwest. Next lift the right foot, gather it to the side of the left foot with the heel landing and toe pointing upward. Simultaneously, the left hand moves to the left and downward, drawing a half circle to the front of the left abdomen. The palm faces down. The right vertical palm in front of the abdomen moves upward in a curve. The right forearm rises upward diagonally in front of the forehead with the palm facing forward and upward. The two hands align in a vertical line. Face southwest. (Figure 88)

Key points: After turning the left foot to point to the southwest, the upper and lower body can start to move. The movements of both arms need to feel round and lively. When the right arm rises, there needs to be the intention of lifting and leading the right foot as it gathers to the left foot. The right shoulder should not rise when the hand moves up. Instead, the shoulder should relax and sink downward. When the right foot gathers closer to the left foot, the body should turn slightly to the right, but it should not be obvious. The upper and lower body need to coordinate.

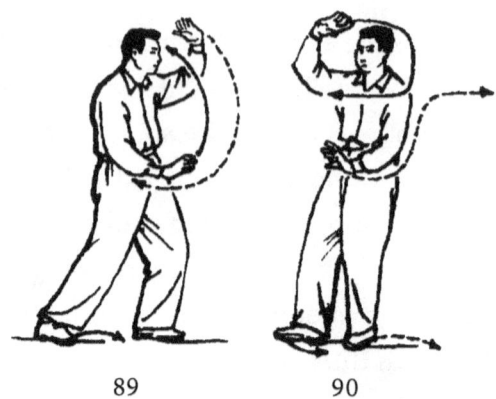

89 90

Movement 3:

The right toe moves to the southeast, and the foot lands flat. With the body following and turning left, look to the southeast. Switch the legs to right substantial and left insubstantial. Next, the left leg takes a step out. The heel lands first and the toe points upward and to the east with a slight southerly direction. Then the right heel pushes and the left leg shifts forward forming a curve, with the foot landing flat and the body moving forward. Simultaneously, the left vertical palm draws a curve from the front of the abdomen upward. The left forearm gradually rises diagonally to the forehead with the palm facing up and forward. The right vertical palm, with the palm facing down, moves to the right and downward in a half circle to the right front of the abdomen. The two hands align in a vertical line. Face southeast. (Figure 89)

Key points: The body and the right foot should turn left simultaneously. After turning, Spirit immediately focuses on the right leg. The rest is the same as Movement 1 of this form.

Movement 4:
This is the same as Movement 2 of this form. The key points are the same as well. (Figure 90)

34. Single Whip (Figure 91)

35. Lift Hand (Figures 92-93)

36. High Pat on Horse (Figure 94)

These 3 arrangements form a sequence. Movement 1 is Single Whip. Movements 2 and 3 are Lift Hand, and movement 4 is High Pat on Horse.

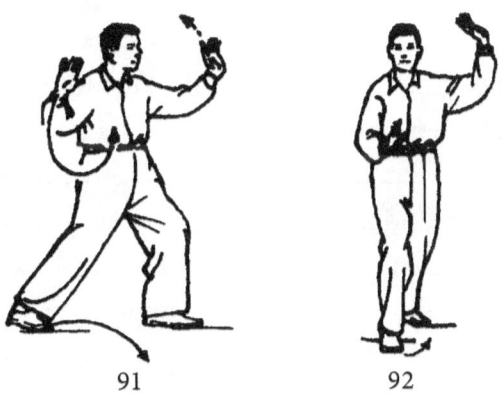

91   92

Movement 1:
The right toe turns southeast and lands flat with the body turning to the left at the same time and looking to the southeast. The legs become right substantial and left insubstantial. Immediately following, the left leg steps out forward with the heel landing first and the toe pointing

upward. Simultaneously, the left hand rises up, the right hand drops, and the two vertical palms are positioned at the height of the shoulder as if pushing a ball. Afterward, the right heel pushes and the left leg shifts forward forming a curve until the left foot lands flat as the body still moves forward. The two hands separate to the left and right, with the left hand at shoulder height and the right hand slightly lower. Face east with a slight southerly direction. (Figure 91)

Key points: When the left hand is rising, it feels like it is coming from the chest up and outward with the intention of lifting and leading the left leg stepping forward. The rest of the key points are the same as the 4th form (Single Whip) Movement number 3.

Movement 2:

Look to the south. Using the left heel as the axle, the left toe turns to the southeast. The foot lands flat and the legs change to left substantial and right insubstantial. Then the right foot lifts and gathers closer to the left foot with the right toe touching the ground next to the left foot. While the right foot is lifting, both hands move with it. The right vertical palm moves to the right and down, drawing a half circle to the right front of the abdomen. The fingers point forward. The left hand is above the forehead with the palm facing up. Face south. (Figure 92)

Key points: This is the same as the 5th form (Lift Hand) Movement 4. The key points are the same as well.

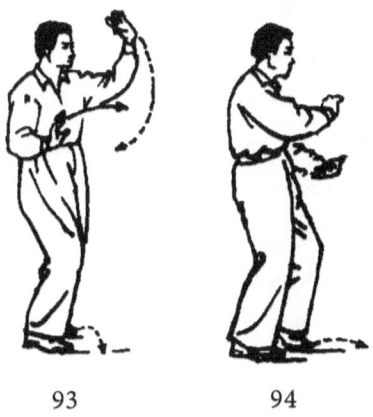

93   94

Movement 3:

The direction stays the same. The right leg steps forward with the heel landing first and the toe pointing upward. At the same time, the right vertical palm rises slightly. Next, the left heel pushes and the right leg shifts forward forming a curve until the foot lands flat as the body moves forward. The left heel pushes, with the right vertical palm slowly extending forward. Face south. (Figure 93)

Key points: When the right leg is stepping forward, it needs to maintain body stability. When the left heel pushes, the left hand has the intention of lifting the sky. Pay attention to relaxing the shoulder and sinking the elbow. While the right hand pushes forward, it needs to have the intention of sinking. The movement, from the foot, to the leg, to the waist, to expressing in the fingers needs to be continuous.

Movement 4:

Look to the east. The right toe turns to the southeast and then lands flat. At the same time, the body turns slightly to the left and the legs change to right substantial and left insubstantial.

Next, the left hand extends slightly forward and toward the east, before dropping down in a curve to the front of the abdomen with the palm turned inwards and eventually up. At the same time, the right vertical palm gathers close to the side of the right ribs, moves forward and presses slightly downward to the front of the chest. With the palm at chest height and facing down, the two palms face each other. Each arm forms a half circle. Simultaneously, the body continues to turn left to face east. While the two arms are moving, the left foot lifts and gathers to the side of the right foot with the left toe touching the ground. (Figure 94)

Key points: The movement of both arms is directed by both sides of the chest. The whole body must coordinate and synchronize. While the body is turning, do not forget the requirement of folding.

37. Left Taming Tiger (Figures 95.1, 95.2, 96)

38. Right Kick (Figures 97-98)

These two arrangements together form a sequence. Movement 1 and 2 are Left Taming Tiger. Movements 3 and 4 are Right Kick.

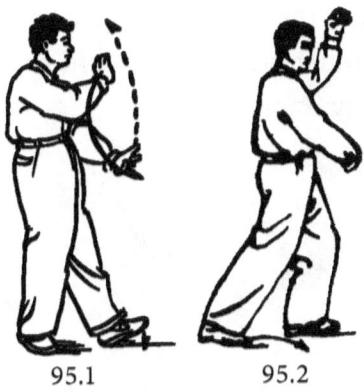

95.1   95.2

Movement 1:

Look to the northeast. The body turns slightly to the left. The left foot steps out to the northeast, with the toe pointing up and the heel landing on the ground. (Figure 95.1) Next, the right heel pushes and the left leg shifts forward forming a curve, with the left foot landing flat and the body shifting forward. The legs are still right substantial and left insubstantial. At the same time, both hands move, with the left hand moving up and forward and forming a fist with the palm facing down in front of the forehead. The right hand drops from the front of the chest to the front of the abdomen. The right forearm rotates outwards and feels full, while the right hand forms a fist with the palm facing up. The two palms face each other vertically. While the two hands are forming a fist, turn to the right, looking toward the southeast. (Figure 95.2)

Key points: When the left hand is moving up, the left chest should have the intention of sinking. After the completion of the form, the left fist needs to have a sinking intention. When the right hand drops, the right forearm needs to have the intention of expansion and fullness and feel connected to the front leg, so that Jin has a source.

At the same time, the abdomen needs to be relaxed and open. The body must not lean forward or back. Be sure to maintain the Body Principles.

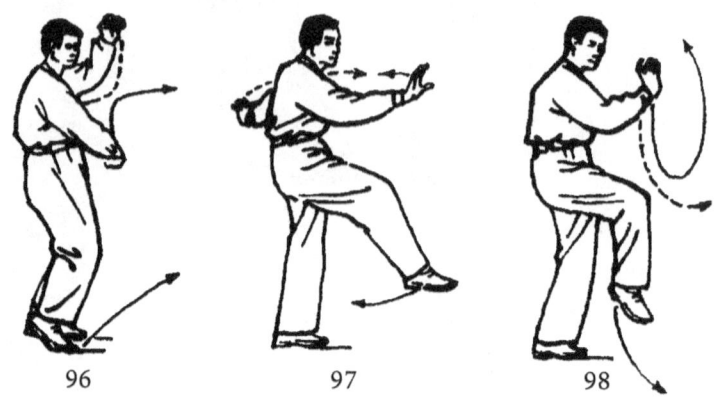

96   97   98

Movement 2:
The legs change to left substantial and right insubstantial. The right leg lifts and gathers next to the side of the left foot with the toe touching the ground. Face southeast. (Figure 96)

Key points: When the right foot is moving, the body and the hands maintain the same posture. The Body Principles stay the same. The transformation of substantial and insubstantial happens internally.

Movement 3:
Look to the southeast. Lift the right leg. At the same time, the right fist rises and the left fist drops. When the two fists are at shoulder height, turn to vertical palms. The right foot lifts and kicks to the southeast to the height of the knee. When kicking, the two vertical palms separate and move to the left and right with the right hand at shoulder height and the left hand slightly lower. The right arm moves in the same

direction as the right leg kicks. The left leg continues to be curved and gathered. (Figure 97)

Key points: While the right fist is rising, it should have the intention of lifting and leading the right leg. The whole body needs to have the intention to gather and remain connected. When the right foot begins to kick, the left leg needs to support and direct the right foot as it extends outward. The top of the right foot should be in a neutral position. The up and down movement of the two fists needs to move from the transformation of the chest energy. The Body Principles remain the same.

Movement 4:
The left and right vertical palms come together in front of the chest at shoulder height. The right hip does not move. The right calf drops down, the toe points down and the heel gathers close to the left knee. Face southeast. (Figure 98)

Key points: When the arms and legs are moving, the whole body needs to have the intention of gathering inwards and staying connected. The two hands and the right leg need to have the intention of embracing the left leg. This is what is called "three embracing the one."

39. Right Taming Tiger (Figures 99.1, 99.2, 100)

40. Left Kick (Figures 101-102)

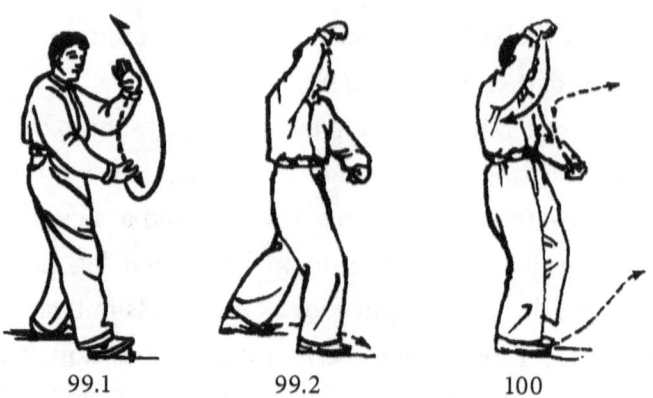

99.1   99.2   100

These two arrangements form a sequence. Movement 1 and 2 are Right Taming Tiger. Movement 3 and 4 are Left Kick.

Movements 1, 2, 3 and 4 are similar to the 37th form (Left Taming Tiger) and the 38th form (Right Kick). The key points are also similar, though the left and right movements are reversed, and the direction and angle are different. In this sequence, Right Taming Tiger, the right foot steps to the southeast and one faces northeast. The right foot kicks to the northeast. (Figures 99.1, 99.2, to 102)

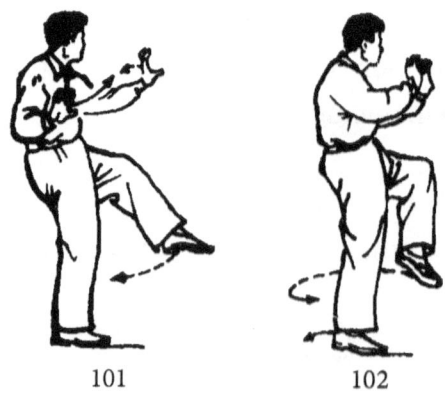

101   102

41. Turn Around and Left Heel Kick (Figures 103-104)

42. Single Whip (Figure 105)

43. Skip and Punch Down (Figure 106)

These 3 arrangements form a sequence. Movements 1 and 2 are Turn Around and Left Heel Kick. Movement 3 is Single Whip. Movement 4 is Skip and Punch Down.

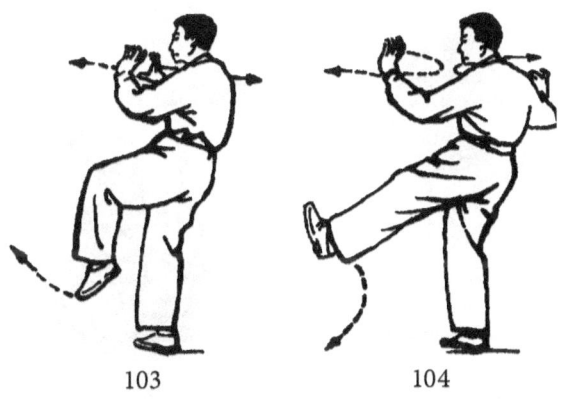

103   104

Movement 1:
Using the right heel as the axle, the body turns left 180 degrees, and faces west. (Figure 103)

Key points: Before turning, the left foot drops to the back side of the right heel with the toe touching the ground. While moving, the left chest should feel insubstantial. Use the right waist eye to lift the left waist eye.

Movement 2:

The left toe points up. Use the left heel to express force, kicking forward. The height should not exceed the lower abdomen. At the same time, the left and right vertical palms separate to the left and right, with the left hand at shoulder height and the right hand slightly lower. The direction of the left arm and the left kick align. Face west. (Figure 104)

Key points: Just before the kick, the body needs to have the intention of gathering inward and staying connected. While kicking, the right leg should support the movement of the left leg, and the upper and lower body need to coordinate with each other while maintaining the Body Principles.

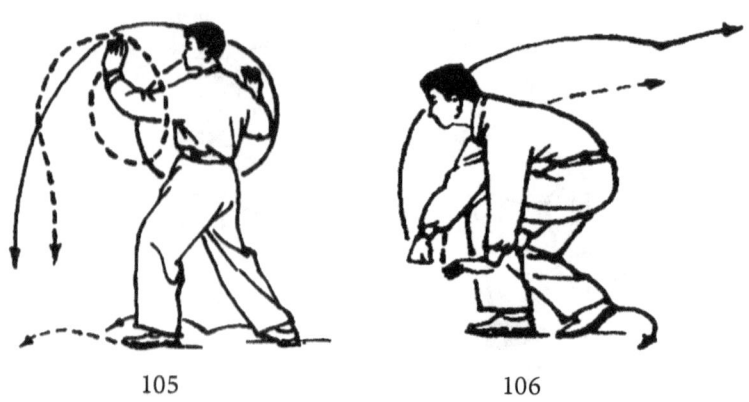

105   106

Movement 3:

The left foot moves forward, landing on the ground heel first. Simultaneously, the two vertical palms come together in front of the chest as if to push a ball. Next, the right heel pushes and the left leg shifts forward forming a curve. The left foot lands flat and the body moves forward. The legs are still right substantial and left insubstantial. While the right heel pushes, the two vertical palms separate left and right forming Single Whip. (Figure 105)

Key points: Land the left heel on the ground. When the two hands gather together, they need to coordinate and follow each other. All other key points are the same as the 4th form Single Whip, Movements 2 and 3. Only the direction and angle are different.

Movement 4:

Skip and Punch Down: Look to the west. The left vertical palm drops to the side of the left hip and then rises, moves forward and downward, drawing a circle, and gathers to the side of the left hip, with the palm facing down. Simultaneously, the right vertical palm rises to the side of the right ear and then first goes forward, and downward and then backward drawing a circle. The right hand changes to a fist at the right hip and then rises up to the side of the right ear. While the two arms are drawing circles, the legs are left substantial and right insubstantial. Next, the right foot steps forward, landing flat next to the left foot. The legs change to right substantial and left insubstantial when the left heel steps forward. The left leg shifts forward forming a curve and the foot lands flat, with the toe pointing to the west. The legs change again to left substantial and right insubstantial. Then the right leg steps forward half a step with the toe landing at the right back side of the left foot. Next the body leans forward and, bending both knees, the body lowers down. When moving downward, the right fist passes by the side of the right ear to the front of the chest and punches down between the front of the legs with the palm facing inward and down. At the same time, the left palm presses down from the side of the left hip to the side of the calf, with the fingers pointing forward. (Figure 106)

Key points: The movement of the arms is directed by both sides of the chest. While stepping, the legs need to transform continuously between substantial and insubstantial. When punching down, the abdomen and back need to be relaxed and open so Qi can stick to the back, sink down, and pass though the buttocks to reach the upper thighs. The waist and leg connect while the body is leaning forward. Stay centered with the eyes looking forward and not down. In this sequence each movement should be connected, and the movement should be continuous, with the upper and lower body coordinated.

44. Turn, Double Rise

(Figures 107.1, 107.2, 108.1, 108.2)

45. Step Back Taming Tiger

(Figures 109.1, 109.2, 110)

These two forms together form a sequence. Movements 1 and 2 are Turn, Double Rise. Movements 3 and 4 are Step Back Taming Tiger.

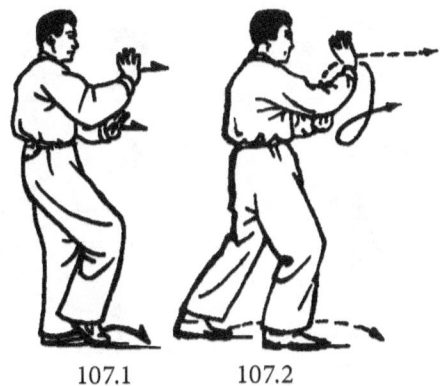

107.1   107.2

Movement 1:

Straighten the body. Using the left heel as the axle, turn around to the right. The left toe turns inward 135 degrees, lands flat and becomes substantial. During the turn, the right fist rises to the face, then drops to the front of the chest and the palm becomes vertical. Simultaneously, the left vertical palm rises to the front of the chest. The right hand is higher and the left lower. The right toe touches the ground while turning and ends up pointing east. (Figure 107.1)

The right leg steps out with the heel landing first. Next, the left heel pushes, the right leg shifts forward forming a curve with the foot landing flat and the body moves forward. The two hands push forward slowly. Face east. (Figure 107.2)

Key points: When straightening the body, Spirit needs to focus on the left leg. While the body turns around to the right, the torso, hand and step need to coordinate with each other. When the right hand lifts, it needs to the have downward intention. After turning, use the left leg to support the right foot as it steps forward and slightly to the right before landing. Other key points are the same as the 3rd form (Right Lan Zha Yi) Movement 3.

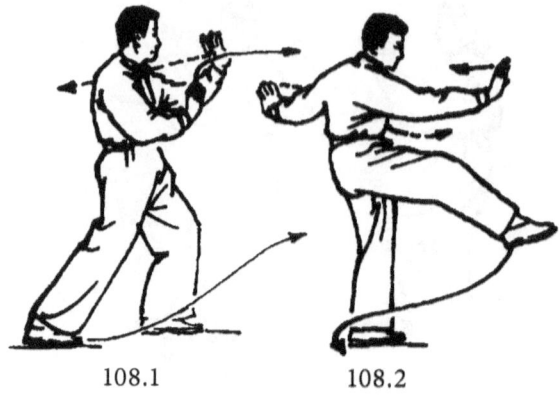

108.1   108.2

Movement 2:

Look to the east. The right toe turns slightly to the outside and the foot lands flat. Next, the legs change to right substantial and left insubstantial. The left leg takes a big step forward, and the heel lands first. While the left leg is stepping forward, the left hand rises to shoulder height, and the right hand draws a curve downward to the height of the chest. Afterward, the right heel pushes and the left leg shifts forward in a curve with the left foot landing flat and the body moving forward while the two vertical palms push forward slowly. (Figure 108.1)

The left toe turns slightly outward and then lands flat. The legs change to left substantial and right insubstantial. The right leg lifts. At the same time, the right hand rises to the same height as the left hand, and the right foot points forward (east) and kicks. Simultaneously, the two hands separate to the left and right. The right hand is at shoulder height, with the left hand slightly lower. The right arm and right leg are aligned and point to the same direction. The right hand has the intention of striking the top of the foot. Still face east. (Figure 108.2)

Key points: When the left hand lifts in Figure 108.1, it needs to have the intention of rising from the chest and coordinating with the left foot when it steps. Other key points are the same as the 2nd form (Left Lan Zha Yi) Movement 3.

Just before lifting, the right foot in figure 108.2, needs to transfer Jin with the tailbone standing. When the right foot lifts, the body needs to remain centered and cannot lean forward or backward. When raising the right hand, the intention needs to come from the chest. While kicking, the top of the right foot needs to have the Jin of Ward Off. Maintain the Body Principles.

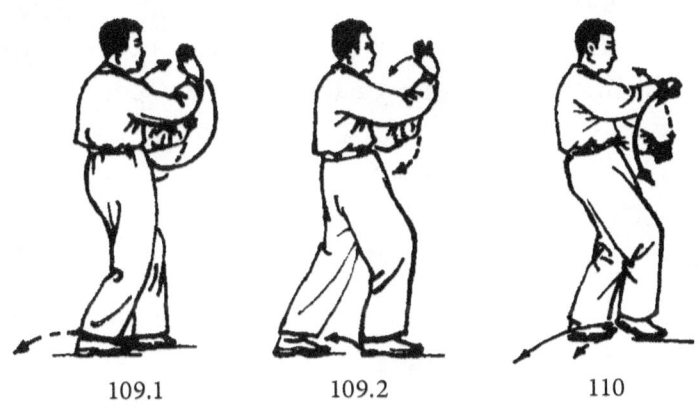

109.1   109.2   110

Movement 3:
The right leg steps back and drops to the left side of the left heel. The toe points east. At the same time, both hands gather to the front of the chest with the right hand at shoulder height and the left hand at the height of the abdomen. (Figure 109.1)

The legs change to right substantial and left insubstantial. The left foot takes a step back, and the toe points to the northeast. Next, the two legs change to left substantial and right insubstantial and the body moves backward. The right toe points up, and the hands move from the front downward and inward and then upward to the front of the chest. Next, the left heel pushes, the right leg shifts forward in a curve with the foot landing flat, and the body moves forward. The legs are still left substantial and right insubstantial. When the left heel pushes, the two vertical palms push forward slowly, with the right hand at shoulder height and the left hand at the height of the abdomen. Face east. (Figure 109.2)

Key points: When stepping back, attention needs to be paid to the exchanges of insubstantial and substantial. The left leg, when stepping back, should not feel extended. The left leg needs to be curved. When the body shifts back, the two hands draw curves moving downward and inward and need the intention of rolling back. Other key points are the same as the 3rd form (Right Lan Zha Yi) Movement 3. Only the direction and angle are different.

Movement 4:
The right leg gathers back and the toe touches down at the side of the left foot. At the same time, the body moves backward. The legs are still left substantial and right insubstantial. Both hands form a fist and gather backward with the body. The left fist has the palm facing up and gathers to the front of the abdomen. The palm of the right fist faces down and gathers to the front of the chest. The palms of the fists face each other, and each of the two arms forms a half circle. Face east. (Figure 110)

Key points: When the right hand is moving, pay attention to sinking the elbow. When the left hand is moving, the left arm has the intention of expanding outward. The upper and lower body need to coordinate. When stepping back, do not lose the forward intention. Continue to maintain the Body Principles.

46. Step Back Left Kick (Figures 111-112)

47. Turn Around Right Heel Kick (Figures 113-114)

48. Step Forward, Parry, Repulse and Punch
(Figure 115.1, 115.2)

These 3 forms together form a sequence. Movements 1 and 2 are Step Back Left Kick, Movement 3 is Turn Around Heel Kick, and Movement 4 is Step Forward, Parry, Repulse and Punch.

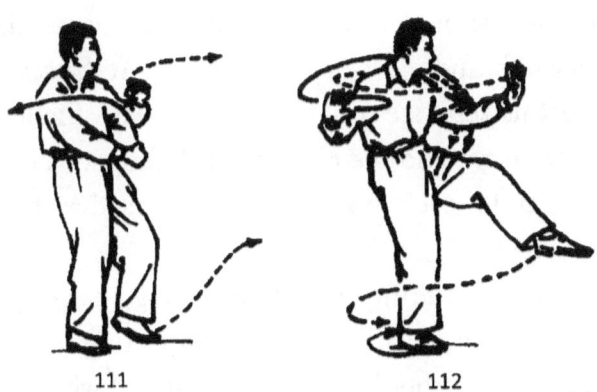

111   112

Movement 1:

The right leg takes a step back and lands flat with the toe pointing to the southeast. The legs change to right substantial and left insubstantial. The body shifts backward, and the left leg gathers backward with the toe touching down at the side of the right foot. When the body is moving back and the left leg is gathering back, the left fist draws a curve upward to the height of the chest, and the right fist draws a curve downward to the front of the abdomen. The two palms of the fists face each other, and the two arms form a half circle. Face east. (Figure 111)

Key points: While stepping back, do not lose the forward intention. At the same time, the two sides of the chest need to direct the curve drawn by the two hands. Pay attention to the folding of the body and the transformation of energy. The body should not lean forward or backward.

Movement 2:

Both fists lift to shoulder height and change to vertical palms. The left leg lifts, and the left foot kicks east. At the same time, the two palms separate to left and right, with the left hand at shoulder height and the right hand slightly lower. The left arm moves and the left foot kicks to the same direction. Face east. (Figure 112)

Key points: While the two fists are lifting, the body should have the intention of gathering and connecting inward. The top of the left foot should have Ward Off Jin when kicking. Maintain the body principles.

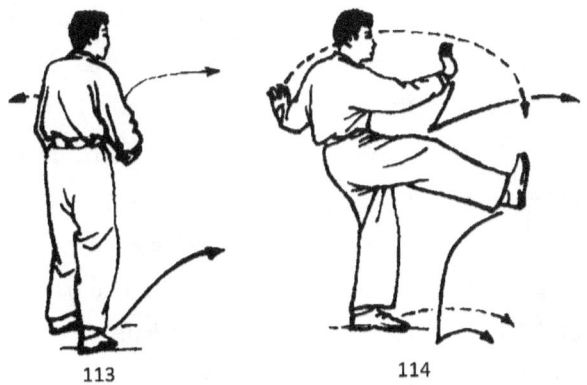

113   114

Movement 3:

The left hip does not move. The calf lowers down with the toe leading, moves down to the right and touches down on the outside of the right foot. At the same time, the two palms gather back to the front of the chest as though preparing to push a ball. Next, using the right foot as the axle, the body and left foot turn 270 degrees to the right together to face northeast. The right heel lands flat, and the two vertical palms turn with the body. Next, the left foot steps out to the northeast, and the heel lands first. The two palms press downward to the front of the abdomen with the fingers pointing forward. Both arms curve slightly. At the same time, the right heel pushes, the left leg shifts forward forming a curve, and the left foot lands flat as the body moves forward. Face northeast. (Figure 113)

The two legs change to left substantial and right insubstantial. The right leg lifts and, at the same time, the two vertical palms lift to shoulder height. Next, the right toe lifts. Use the heel kick to the east at the height of the crotch. Simultaneously, the two vertical palms separate to the left and right with the right hand at shoulder height and the left hand slightly lower. The right arm and the right kick are aligned to the same direction. Face east. (Figure 114)

Key points: Dropping the left calf needs to coordinate with the two hands, gathering back with the body intention of gathering and connecting. While turning the body, the hand and the foot need to move as one, with the body remaining centered. When pressing down, the backs of both hands need to have rising intention. While doing the heel kick, the body needs to keep centered.

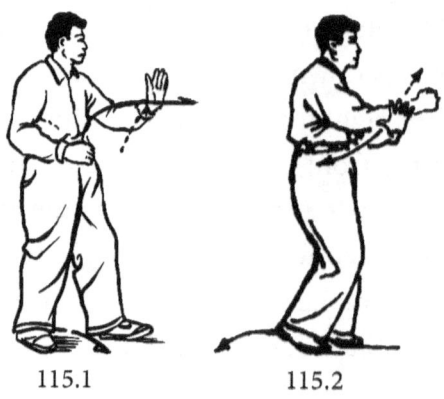

115.1   115.2

Movement 4:
Look to the east. As the right leg lowers, the right foot steps to the right front side of the left foot, and the toe points to the southeast. Simultaneously, the right vertical palm drops to the side of the right hip and the left vertical palm draws a curve upward to the front of the face. (Figure 115.1)

The two legs change to right substantial and left insubstantial. The left leg steps forward with the heel landing first, and next the left leg shifts forward forming a curve. The foot lands flat as the body moves forward. The legs change to left substantial and right insubstantial. The right foot moves forward half a step, and the toe lands next to the side of the left heel. While the left foot is stepping up, the left vertical palm draws a curve from above forward and curves down to the front of the abdomen. Then the right hand forms a fist. When the right foot follows up half a step, the right fist punches slowly forward on top of the left hand, with the palm facing to the left forming a vertical fist at chest height. Face east. (Figure 115.2)

Key points: After the right leg steps forward, Spirit needs to focus on the upper thigh before the left foot can step up. The movement of the two hands needs to be directed by the chest. The rest of the key points are the same as the 11th form (Step Forward, Parry, Repulse and Punch) Movement 4.

49. Withdraw and Push (Figures 116-119)

Movements 1, 2, 3 and 4 are the same as the 12th form (Withdraw and Push) four Movements. The key points are the same as well. (Figures 116-119)

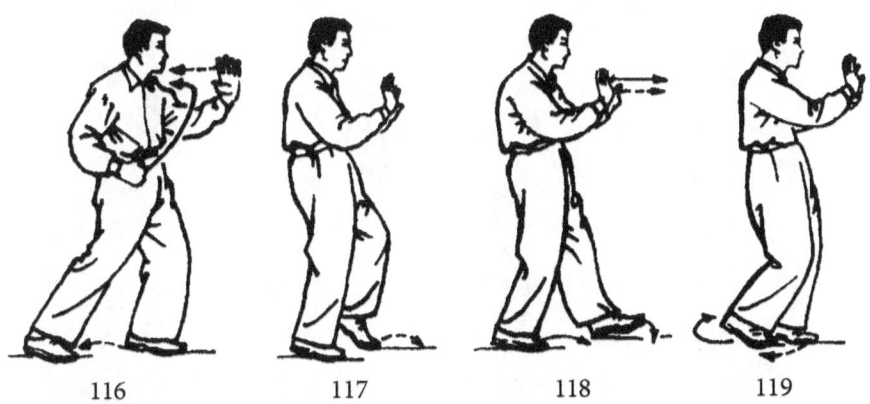

| 116 | 117 | 118 | 119 |

50. Carry Tiger, Push Mountain (Figures 120-123)

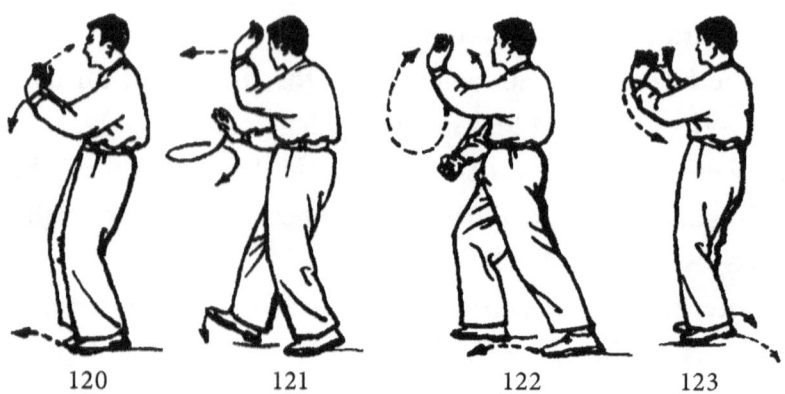

120   121   122   123

Movements 1, 2, 3 and 4 are the same as the 13th form's four movements (Carry Tiger, Push Mountain). The key points are the same as well. (Figures 120-123)

51. Play the Guitar (Figure 124)

52. Right Lan Zha Yi (Figure 125-127)

These two forms together form a sequence. Movement 1 is Play the Guitar. Movements 2, 3 and 4 are right Lan Zha Yi.

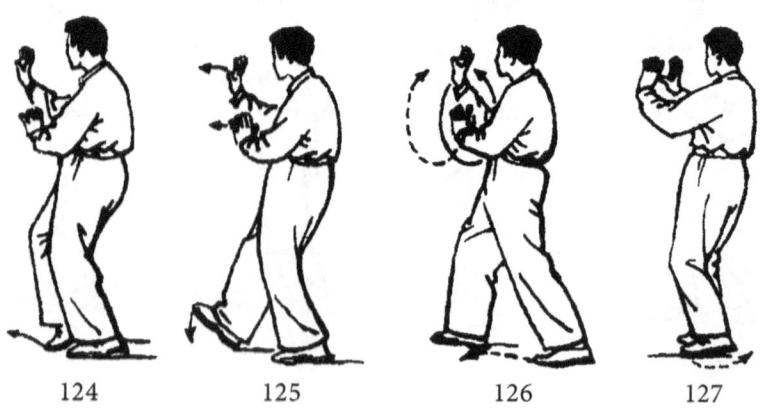

124   125   126   127

Movement 1 is the same as the 14th form (Play the Guitar) Movement 1. The key points are the same. Only the direction and angle are different. This form faces northwest. (Figure 124)

Movement 2 is the same as the 15th form (Right Lan Zha Yi) Movement 2. The key points are the same. Only the direction and angle are different. This form faces northwest. (Figure 125)

Movements 3 and 4 and the 3rd form (Right Lan Zha Yi) Movements 3 and 4 are the same. The key points are the same as well. Only the direction and angle are different. This form faces northwest. (Figures 126, 127)

53. Diagonal Single Whip (Figures 128-130)

54. Down Posture (Figure 131)

These two forms together form a sequence. Movements 1, 2 and 3 are Diagonal Single Whip. Movement 4 is Down Posture.

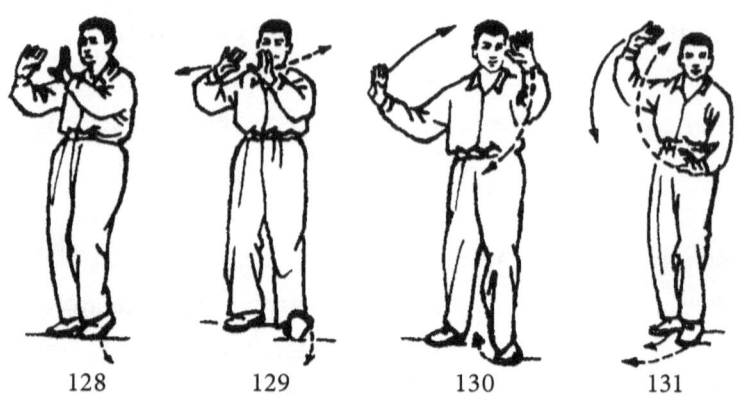

Movements 1, 2 and 3 are the same as the 4th form (Single Whip) Movements 1, 2 and 3. The key points are the same as well. Only the direction and angle are different. This form steps to the south with the chest facing southwest. (Figures 128-130)

Movement 4 is the same as the 32nd form (Down Posture) Movement 4. The key points are the same as well. Only the direction and angle are different. This form faces southwest. (Figure 131)

55. Wild Horse Parts Mane (Figures 132-135)

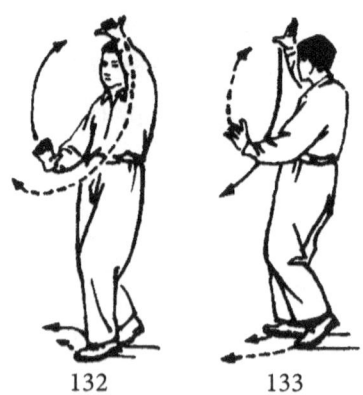

Movement 1:

The body turns slightly to the right, looking to the southwest and the left leg takes a step to the southwest. The heel lands first, and next the left vertical palm moves from in front of the abdomen to the right and up, and then to the left, drawing a curve. Rising to the left forehead, the right vertical palm draws a curve downward in front of the right side of the abdomen. At the same time, the body moves forward. The left leg curves, with the foot landing flat. Next, the left leg becomes substantial and the right insubstantial. The right foot follows, taking a half step with the toe touching down at the side of the left heel. Face southwest. (Figure 132)

Key points: When the left leg steps up, the body must be stable. Focus Spirit on the right leg. The movement of both arms needs to be round and lively. Before the right foot moves up, the legs need to finish changing from substantial to insubstantial. While the right foot is moving up, the body must not lean forward or backward. The abdomen needs to be relaxed.

Movement 2:

Look to the northwest. The right leg takes a step to the northwest with the heel landing first. The body turns slightly to the right. The left vertical palm draws a curve down to the front of the left abdomen. Starting from the left, the right vertical palm moves up from the front of the abdomen and then to the right in a curve, to the right front of the forehead. While both hands are drawing the curve, the body moves forward with the right leg curved and the foot lands flat. The legs change to right substantial and left insubstantial. The left foot follows up half a step with the toe landing to the side of the right heel. Face northwest. (Figure 133)

Key points: This is the same as Movement 1 of this form. Only the direction and angle are different. The left and right movements are opposite.

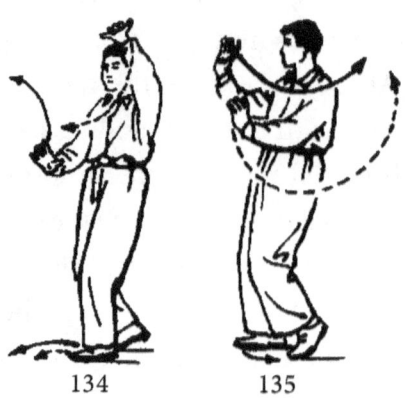

134   135

Movement 3:

The explanation is the same as for Movement 1 of this form, except that the left leg steps forward and the body turns slightly to the left. The key points are the same. (Figure 134)

Movement 4:

Look to the west. The right leg takes a step to the west. The heel lands first. At the same time, the left vertical palm draws a curve downward, and the right vertical palm moves upward from the front of the abdomen. It looks like right Lan Zha Yi. Next, the right leg forms a curve with the right foot landing flat. The body moves forward, and the legs change to right substantial and left insubstantial. The left foot steps forward one half step with the toe touching down to the left side of the right foot. While the left foot is stepping forward, the two vertical palms push out slowly. The right hand is in the front at shoulder height and the left hand is behind at the height of the abdomen. Face west. (Figure 135)

Key points: The two arms moving in a curve need to coordinate with the right leg stepping up. During the following step, the right leg needs to have Spirit focused and stable. The body must not lean forward or backward when the two hands are pushing forward. The chest and back need to open and relax with the Qi sinking down.

56. Single Whip (Figures 136-139)

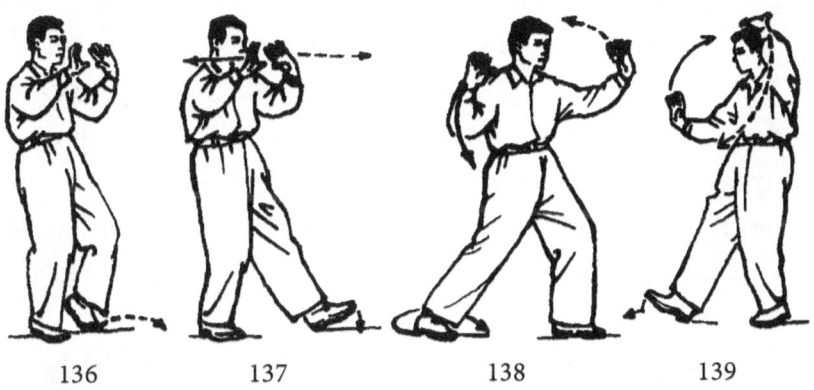

| 136 | 137 | 138 | 139 |

Movement 1:

The left foot moves behind and to the left with the toe touching the ground. Next, using the right heel as the axle, the body and the right toe turn left 135 degrees to the southeast. The legs are still right substantial and left insubstantial. The left vertical palm turns with the body and draws a curve downward to the front of the abdomen and then upward to be even with the right hand, which is in front of the chest at shoulder height. The hands are positioned as if pushing a ball. (Figure 136)

Key points: The movement of the left hand is directed by the left chest and is coordinated with the turning of the body. The sensation is round and lively.

Movements 2 and 3 are the same as the 4th form (Single Whip) Movements 2 and 3. The key points are the same as well. (Figures 137, 138)

Movement 4:

The left toe turns inward and lands flat. At the same time, the body turns to the right 135 degrees to face the southwest. The two legs change to left substantial and right insubstantial. The right leg lifts and turns. The toe turns and points to the west and the heel lands with the toe pointing up. As the body turns, the left hand, with the palm facing up, lifts in front of the forehead. Simultaneously, the right vertical palm drops down to the front of the chest. Face southwest. (Figure 139)

Key points: When the left toe turns inward, the body and toe need to turn together. After turning, immediately focus Spirit on the left leg. The body needs to be stable when the right leg lifts. Maintain the Body Principles. Throughout the entire movement, the body, hands and steps must coordinate properly.

57. Fair Lady Weaves Shuttle (Figures 140.1, 140.2-143)

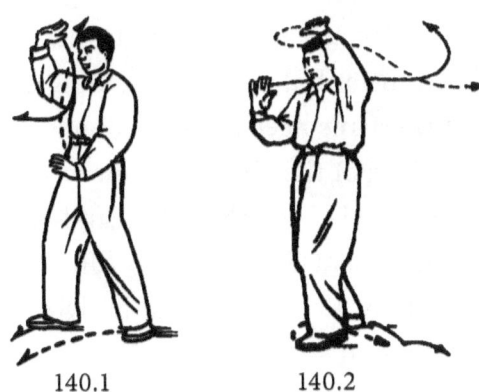

140.1   140.2

Movement 1:

Look to the southwest. The left heel pushes, and the right leg shifts forward to form a curve, with the foot landing flat and the body moving forward.

Simultaneously, the left vertical palm moves to the left and downward and then to the right to draw a curve to the front of the left abdomen. The right vertical palm lifts from in front of the chest to the forehead with the forearm at a diagonal. (Figure 140.1)

The legs change to right substantial and left insubstantial. The left leg takes a big step to the southwest with the heel landing first. Immediately the left leg forms a curve with the foot landing flat and the body shifting forward. The legs change to left substantial and right insubstantial. The right foot moves up half a step with the toe landing next to the side of the left heel. At the same time, the left vertical palm lifts above the left side of the forehead with the left forearm at a diagonal, and the right vertical palm drops down from the side of the right ear to the front of the chest. When the right foot steps up, the right vertical palm slowly pushes forward toward the southwest. Face southwest. (Figure 140.2)

Key points: Pay attention to the transformation of insubstantial to substantial and body folding exchanges. The movement of the arms needs to feel connected and attracted to the two sides of the chest. Do not move too far away. It is important to relax the shoulders and sink the elbows. During the movement all must coordinate appropriately. Maintain the Body Principles. The body should not lean forward or backward.

Movement 2:
Lift the right foot and move it backward to the left side of the left heel with the toe touching the ground. Next, using the left heel as the axle, the body and the left toe turn to the right (southeast) 225 degrees together. Afterward, the right leg steps toward the southeast with the heel landing first. Next, the right leg forms a curve with the foot landing flat and the body shifting forward. After the right foot lands flat, the legs change to right substantial and left insubstantial. The left foot follows up half a step with the toe landing next to the right heel. As the right leg is stepping up, the right vertical palm rises diagonally past the front of the face, to above the forehead. The fingers point to the left. The left vertical palm drops from the side of the left ear to the front of the chest. As the left foot moves half a step up, the left vertical palm slowly pushes forward to the southeast. Face southeast. (Figure 141)

Key points: When the body turns around to the right, maintain the Body Principles and remain stable. Other key points are the same as Movement 1 of this form. Only the left and right movements are opposite, and the angle and direction different.

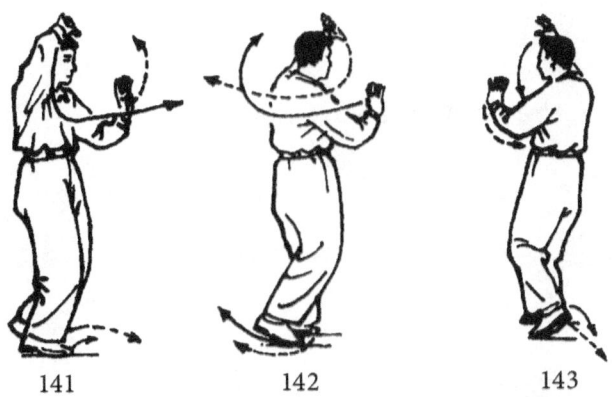

141   142   143

Movement 3:

Look to the northeast. The body turns slightly to the left and the left leg steps up to the northeast with the heel landing first, the body shifting forward and the foot landing flat. The legs change to left substantial and right insubstantial. The right leg moves up half a step with the toe landing next to the side of the left heel. When the left leg is stepping forward, the left forearm (slanted diagonally) rises diagonally in front of the face and stops above the forehead. The right vertical palm drops from the side of the right ear to the front of the chest. As the right foot follows half a step, the right vertical palm pushes forward slowly. Face northeast. (Figure 142)

Key points: This is the same as Movement 1 of this form. Only the direction and angle are different.

Movement 4:

Movement 4 is the same as Movement 2 of this form. Only the direction and angle are different. This movement turns around 225 degrees to the right. The right leg steps to the northwest. The key points are the same. Face northwest. (Figure 143)

58. Play the Guitar (Figure 144)

59. Right Lan Zha Yi (Figures 145-147)

These two forms together form a sequence. Movement 1 is Play the Guitar, Movements 2, 3 and 4 are Right Lan Zha Yi.

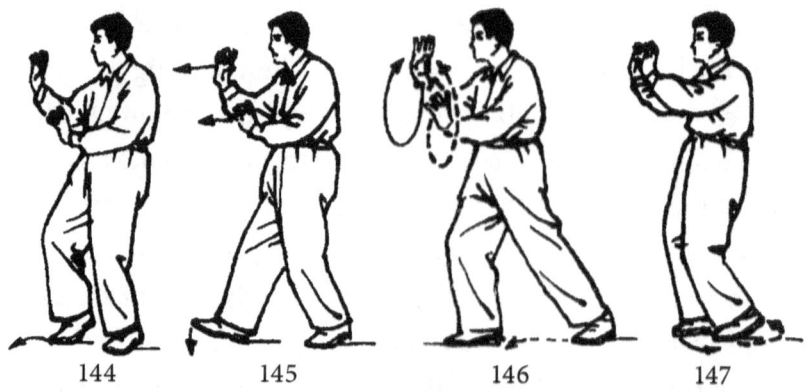

144   145   146   147

Movement 1 is the same as the 14th form (Play the Guitar), and the key points are the same. (Figure 144)

Movements 2, 3 and 4 are the same as the 15th form (Right Lan Zha Yi) Movements 2, 3 and 4, and the key points are the same. (Figures 145-147)

60. Single Whip (Figures 148-150)

61. Down Posture (Figure 151)

These two forms together form a sequence. Movements 1, 2 and 3 are Single Whip, and Movement 4 is Down Posture.

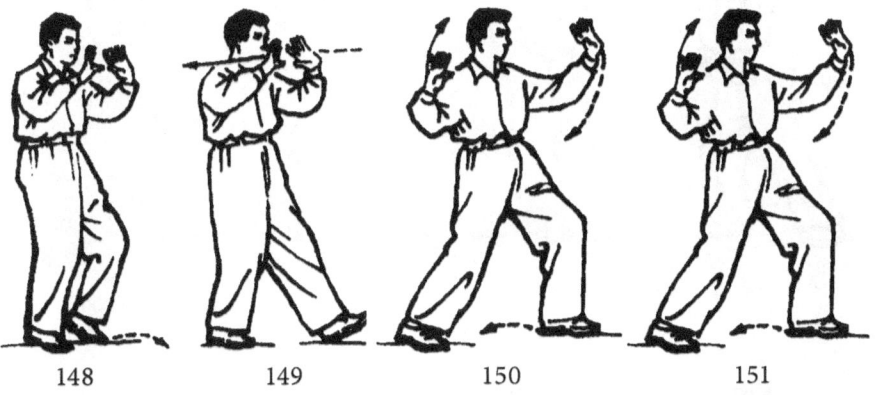

148   149   150   151

Movement 1 is the same as the 16th form (Single Whip) Movement 1, and the key points are the same. (Figure 148)

Movements 2 and 3 are the same as the 4th form (Single Whip), Movement 2 and 3 and the key points are the same. (Figures 149, 150)

Movement 4 is the same as the 31st form (Single Whip) and 32nd form (Down Posture) sequence's Movement 4, and the key points are the same. (Figure 151)

62. Cloud Hands (Figures 152-155)

Movements 1, 2, 3 and 4 and the 33rd form (Cloud Hands) 4 movements are the same, and the key points are the same as well. (Figures 152-155)

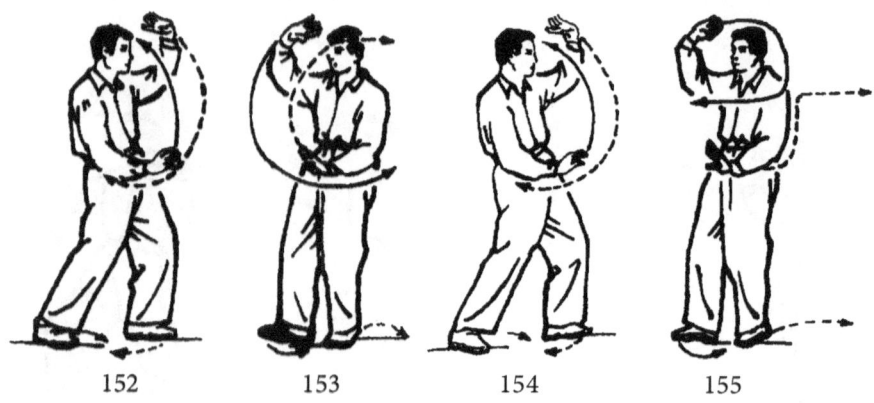

152   153   154   155

63. Single Whip (Figure 156)

64. Down Posture (Figure 157)

65. Rooster Stands on One Leg (Figures 158-159)

These three forms together form a sequence. Movement 1 is Single Whip, Movement 2 is Down Posture and Movements 3 and 4 are Rooster Stands on One Leg.

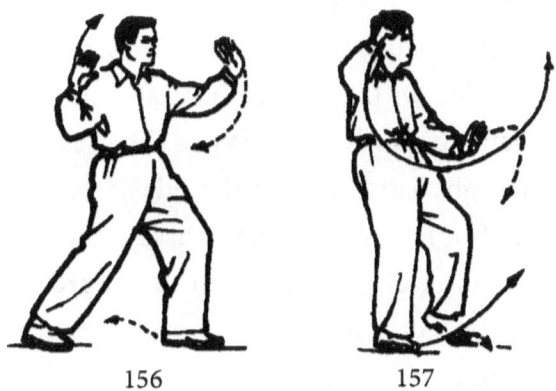

156   157

Movement 1 is the same as the 34th form (Single Whip) Movement 1, and the key points are the same. (Figure 156)

Movement 2 and the 31st form (Single Whip) and 32nd form (Down Posture) sequence's Movement 4 is the same, and the key points are the same as well. (Figure 157)

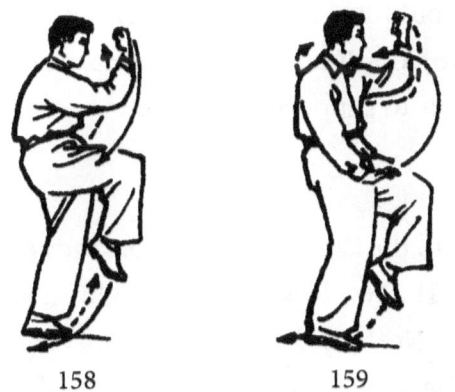

158   159

Movement 3:
Look to the east. The left leg steps forward with the heel landing first and the toe pointing to the east. Next shift the body slowly forward, while at the same time turning slightly

to the left. The left leg is slightly curved with the foot landing flat. The legs change to left substantial and right insubstantial. The right leg lifts with the knee bent and the calf hanging down. The left leg stands alone. When the left leg is stepping forward, the right hand drops to the side of the right hip and forms a fist. The left vertical palm rises slightly. When the right leg lifts, the right fist's palm turns inward and rises to the top of the head. The forearm forms a vertical with the right upper thigh. Simultaneously, the left hand press down from above to the side of the left hip, with the palm facing down and the fingers pointing forward. The left arm is slightly curved. Face east. (Figure 158)

Key points: One must focus Spirit on the left leg and relax the abdomen. The tailbone stands up before lifting the right leg. When lifting the leg, the right foot must have Ward Off energy. At the same time, the movements of the two arms and chest should not be too far apart. The upper and lower body need to coordinate. The body must not lean to either side and needs to support all 8 directions.

Movement 4:
Still looking to the east. The right foot lands flat at the side of the left foot. The two legs change to right substantial and left insubstantial. Next, the left leg lifts to the height of the upper thigh with the knee bent, the calf hanging down and the toe pointing downward. The right leg stands alone. The right fist turns to a vertical palm. The palm presses down toward the side of the right hip with the palm facing downward and the fingers pointing forward. At the same time, the left hand

forms a fist at the side of the left hip with the palm facing inward and rises head high. The forearm forms a vertical with the left thigh. Face east. (Figure 159)

Key points: It is the same as Movement 3 of this sequence, and the key points are the same as well. Only the left and right are reversed.

66. Left Repulse Monkey (Figure 160-163)

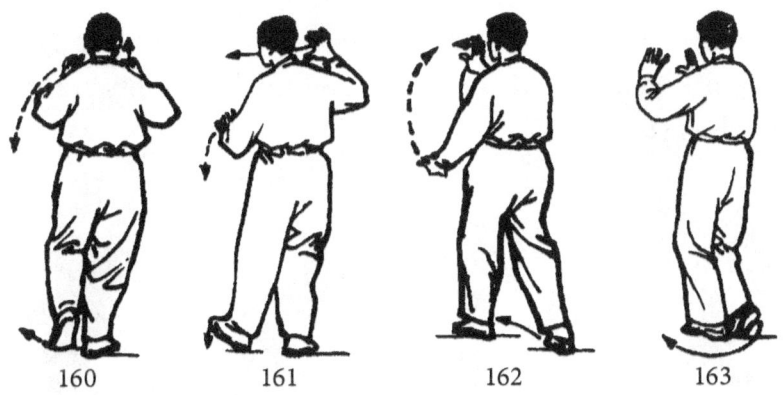

| 160 | 161 | 162 | 163 |

Movement 1:

The left foot drops down with the toe touching down at the back of the right heel. Next using the right foot as the axle, the body and the right toe turn to the left 90 degrees. The legs are still right substantial and left insubstantial. Following the drop of the left foot, the body turns left. The two hands switch to vertical palms and separate to the left and right, first dropping and then moving upward in a curve. When the body turns and faces north, the two hands should be in front of the chest at shoulder height, positioned as though pushing a ball. Face north. (Figure 160)

Key points: Maintain Spirit's focus on the right leg. The movement of the arms needs to be round and lively. The curve drawn by the left hand should be slightly larger and the one drawn by the right hand slightly smaller. The speed of the right hand dropping is slower. After lowering both hands, when the arms start moving upward, they should move together. At the same time, the shoulders need to follow and relax and open the back. Maintain the Body Principles.

Movements 2, 3 and 4 are the same as the 49th form (Left Repulse Monkey) Movement 4, and the key points are the same as well.

67. Right Repulse Monkey (Figures 164-167)

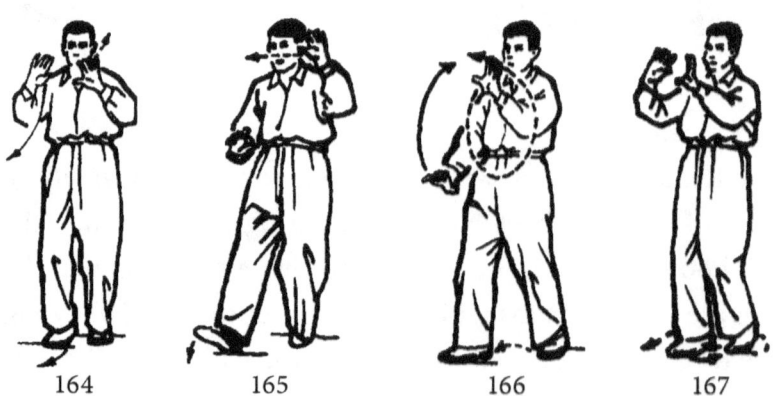

Movements 1, 2, 3 and 4 and the 20th form (Right Repulse Monkey) four movements are the same, and the key points are the same as well. (Figures 164-167)

68. Left Repulse Monkey (Figures 168-171)

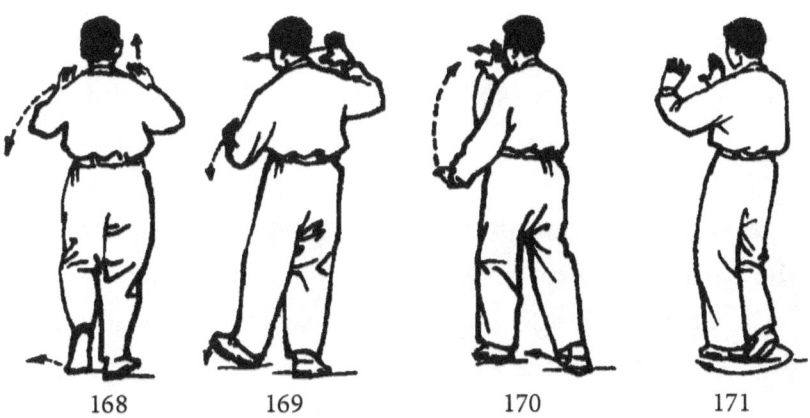

168   169   170   171

Movements 1, 2, 3 and 4 and 21st form (Left Repulse Monkey) four movements are the same, and the key points are the same as well. (Figures 168-171)

69. Right Repulse Monkey (Figures 172-175)

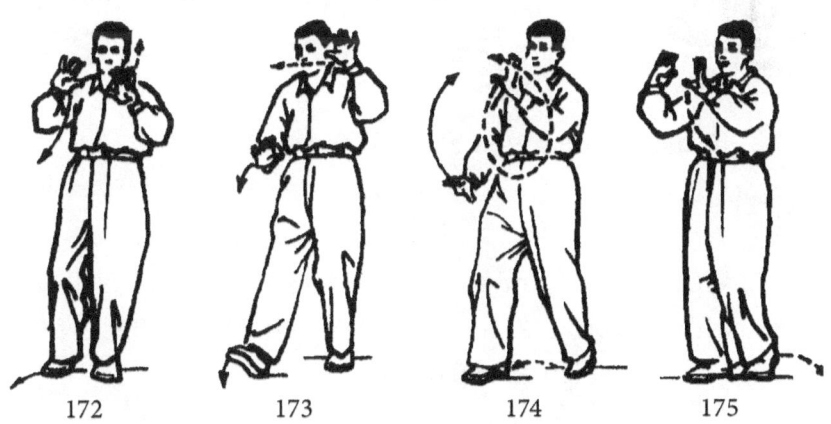

172   173   174   175

Movements 1, 2, 3 and 4 and 20th form (Right Repulse Monkey) four movements are the same and the key points are the same as well. (Figures 172-175)

70. Play the Guitar (Figure 176)

71. White Swan Spreads Wings (Figures 177-179)

These two forms together form a sequence. It is the same as the 23rd form (Play the Guitar) and the 24th form (White Swan Spreads Wings) sequence's four Movements. The key points are the same as well. (Figures 176-179)

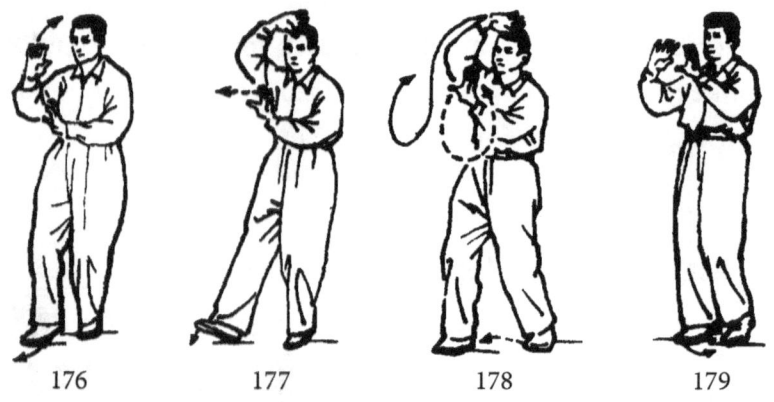

176   177   178   179

72. Brush Knee Twist Step (Figures 180-183)

Movements 1, 2, 3 and 4 are the same as the 7th form (Brush Knee Twist Step) four Movements and the key points are the same as well. (Figures 180-183)

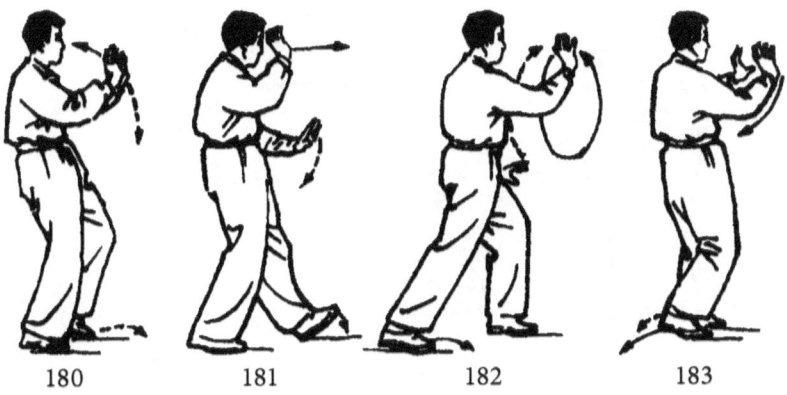

180   181   182   183

73. Play the Guitar (Figure 184)

74. Press Down (Figure 185)

75. Green Dragon Rises Out of Water
(Figure 186.1-186.2)

76. Turn Around (Figures 187.1-187.2)

These four forms together form a sequence. It is the same as the sequence of the 26th form (Play the Guitar), 27th form (Press Down), the 28th form (Green Dragon Rises Out of Water), and the 29th form (Turn Around), and the key points are the same as well. (Figures 184-187)

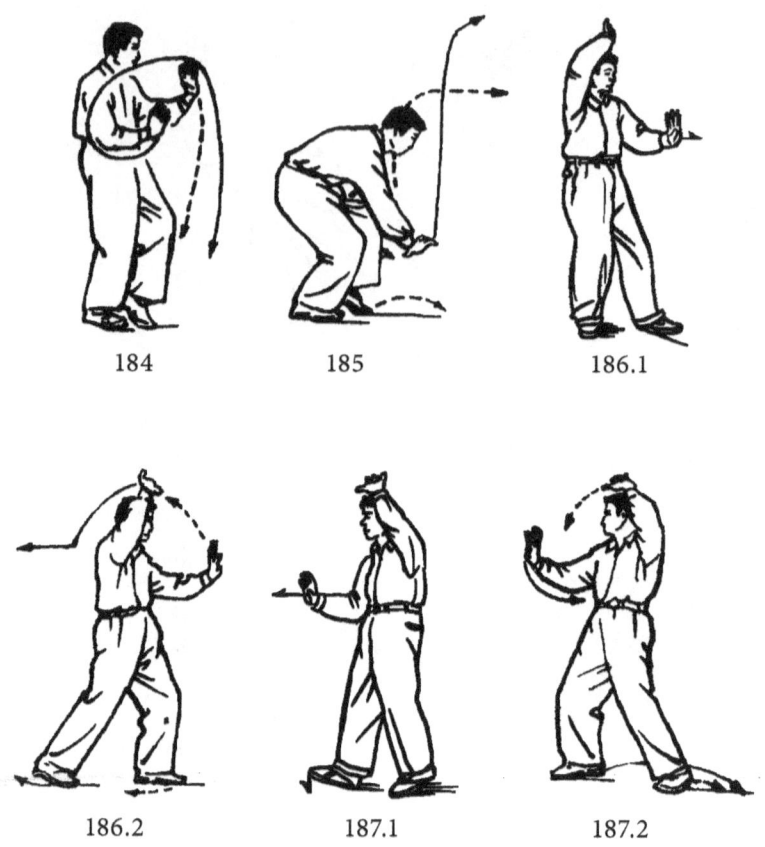

184   185   186.1

186.2   187.1   187.2

77. Three Changing Backs (Figures 188-191)

Movements 1, 2, 3 and 4 are the same as the 30th form (Three Changing Backs) four Movements, and key points are the same as well. (Figures 188-191)

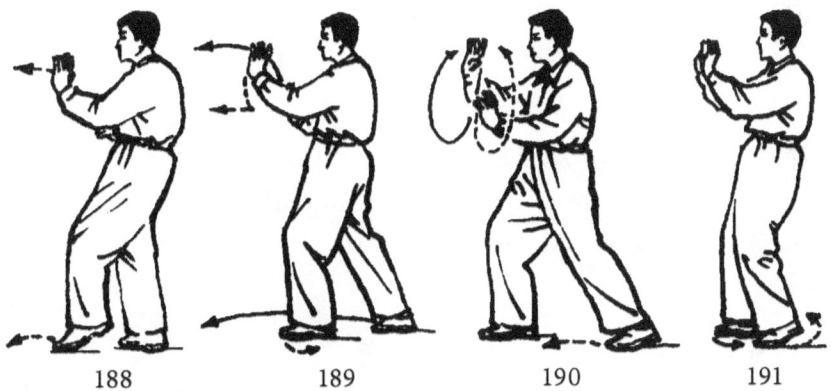

188   189   190   191

78. Single Whip (Figures 192-194)

79. Down Posture (Figure 195)

These two forms together form a sequence. This is the same sequence and the same Movements as the 31st form (Single Whip) and the 32nd form (Down Posture). The key points are the same as well. (Figures 192-195)

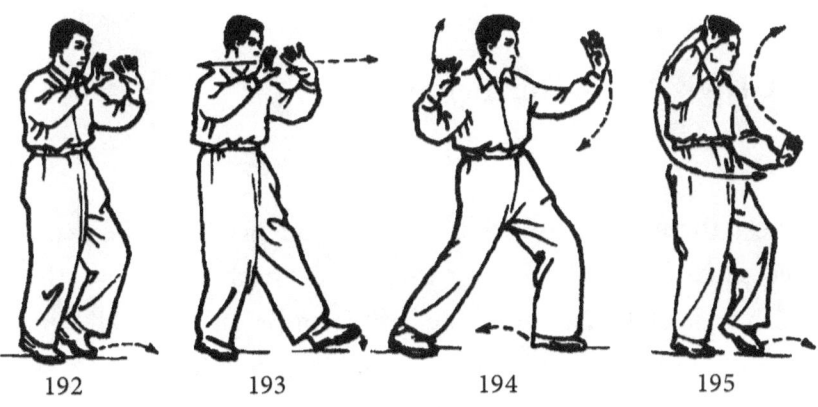

192   193   194   195

80. Cloud Hands (Figures 196-199)

Movements 1, 2, 3 and 4 are the same as the 33rd form (Cloud Hands) four Movements, and the key points are the same as well. (Figures 196-199)

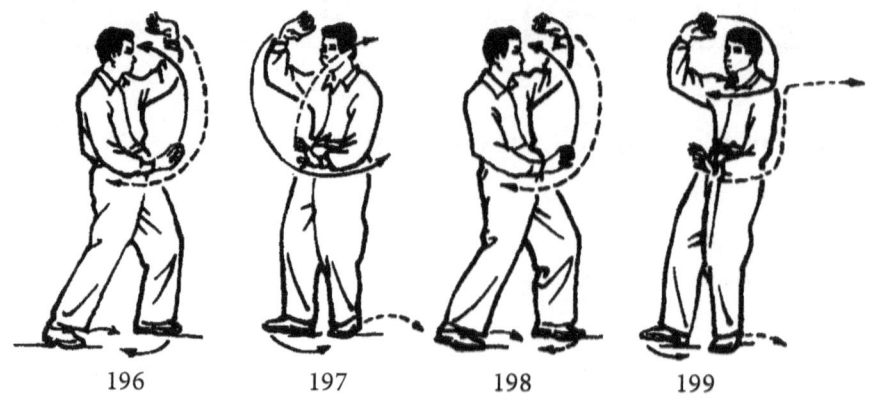

196   197   198   199

81. Single Whip (Figure 200)

82. Lift Hand (Figures 201-202)

83. High Pat on Horse (Figure 203)

These three forms together form a sequence. It is the same sequence and Movements as the 34th form (Single Whip), the 35th form (Lift Hand) and the 36th form (High Pat on Horse), and key points are the same as well. (Figures 200-203)

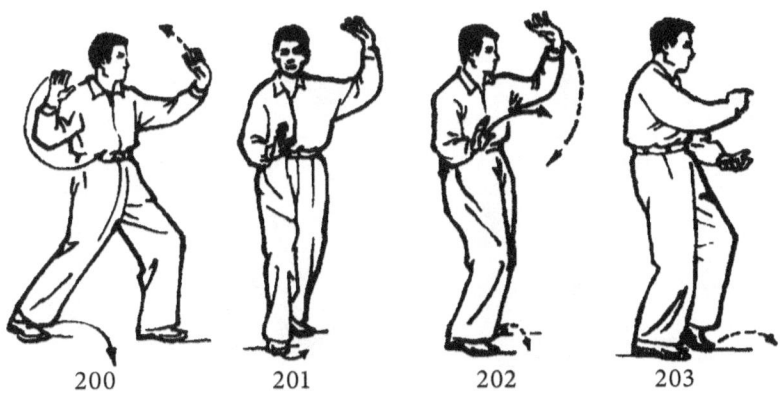

84. Heart Palm (Figures 204.1-204.2)

85. Turn, Cross Lotus Kick (Figures 205.1, 205.2)

86. Step Up, Low Punch (Figures 206.1-206.2)

87. Step Up Right Lan Zha Yi (Figure 207)

These four forms together form a sequence. Movement 1 is Heart Palm, Movement 2 is Turn Cross Lotus Kick, Movement 3 is Step Up, Low Punch and Movement 4 is Step Up Right Lan Zha Yi.

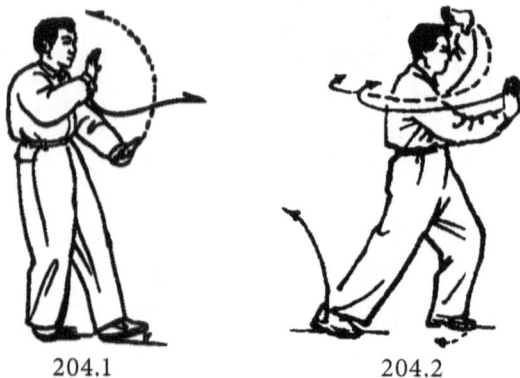

204.1   204.2

Movement 1:

Face the same direction. The left leg steps forward to the east with the heel landing first and the toe pointing up. (Figure 204.1)

Next, the right heel pushes and the left leg shifts forward forming a curve with the foot landing flat and the body shifting forward. The legs are still right substantial and left insubstantial. At the same time, the left hand moves in front of the right hand and up to the forehead. The palm turns to face up. The fingers still point to the right. At the same time, the right elbow drops and the right hand changes to a vertical palm. Following the thrust of the right heel, the right palm slowly pushes out, with the fingers at the height of the shoulder. Face east. (Figure 204.2)

Key Points: Face northwest. After the left foot steps out, the motion of the two arms needs to have the intention of "leading" and "gathering," At the same time, pay attention to relaxing the shoulder and dropping the elbow. Gather before expressing Jin. As the right hand pushes forward, the thrust of the right foot needs to coordinate and move as one. The body should not lean forward or backward.

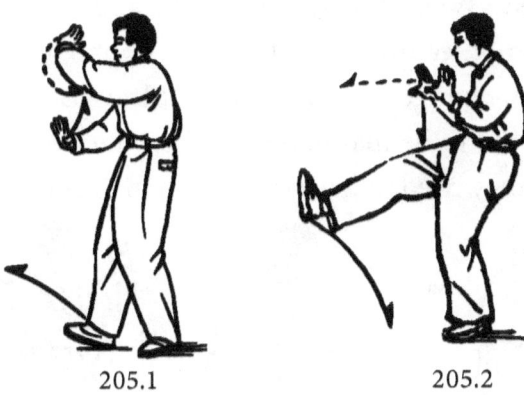

205.1   205.2

Movement 2:

(Turn, Cross Lotus Kick) Using the left heel as the axle, the body and the left toe turn around to the right 135 degrees. Immediately afterward, the left foot lands flat, and the legs change to left substantial and right insubstantial. Look to the west. As the right leg becomes insubstantial, lift the right foot with the toe turned to the west and the heel touching the ground. (figure 205.1)

Next, the right leg lifts with the toe pointing up. From the lower left, sweep around to the upper right with the bottom of the foot facing forward at the height of the knee. The two arms move with the leg motion. The right vertical palm lifts slightly, the left vertical palm drops to the front of the chest, and the two arms cross with the left hand outside. When the right leg is sweeping, the two vertical palms separate to the left and right. The fingertips are at shoulder height. Face west. (Figure 205.2)

Key points: When the body is turning around to the right, up and down must coordinate and move together. After the left foot lands flat, Spirit must focus on the left leg and be stable. When lifting, the right hand needs to have the intention of leading and lifting the right leg. While the right leg is sweeping, the body must not lean back. All Body Principles need to be maintained. When the two hands are separating, they need to have the intention of sinking.

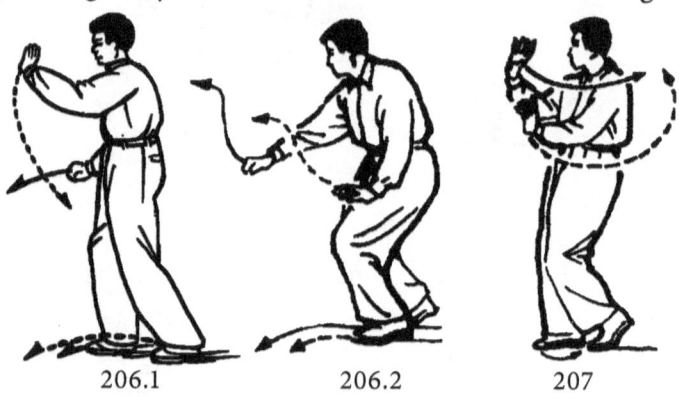

206.1   206.2   207

Movement 3:

(Step Up, Low Punch) Look to the west. The right foot lands flat in front of the right side of the right foot. Immediately the legs change to right substantial and left insubstantial. The right vertical palm drops to the side of the right hip forming a fist with the palm facing down. The left vertical palm moves forward, drawing a curve with the fingers at shoulder height. (Figure 206.1)

The left leg takes a step forward. The heel lands first with the toe pointing to the southwest. Next, the left foot lands flat with the leg slightly curved and the body shifts forward with the motion. The two legs change to left substantial and right insubstantial. The right foot moves up half a step with the toe touching the side of the left heel. While the left leg is stepping up, the left hand moves from the front of the chest downward and sweeps across above the left knee and stops at the side of the left leg, with the fingers pointing forward and the palm facing down. The right fist slowly punches outward. The right foot moves up half a step to the left foot. The palm of the left hand faces down at the height of the crotch. The two arms are slightly bent. The body leans forward slightly. Face west. (Figure 206.2)

Key points: Pay attention to the exchanges of insubstantial and substantial. During the steps, both legs should be able to gather strength. The motion of both arms needs to be directed by the movement of the chest energy. The two shoulders open when the back opens. The Jin of the right fist needs to have a source. Up and down need to coordinate with each other.

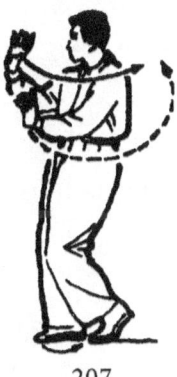

207

Movement 4:

(Step Up Right Lan Zha Yi): Look to the west. Straighten the body. The right leg steps forward with the heel landing first. At the same time both vertical hands rise to the front of the chest. The right hand is higher and in front, with the left hand lower and behind. The right leg lands first with a slight bend, and the body moves forward. The legs change to right substantial and left insubstantial. When the left foot moves up to the right foot, the toe touches the back side of the right heel. While the left foot is moving up, both vertical palms push out slowly. The right hand is at shoulder height and the left hand is at the height of the chest. Face west. (Figure 207)

Key points: When both arms are rising, they need to coordinate with the movement of the right foot. Other key points are the same as the 55th form (Wild Horse Parts Mane) Movement 4.

88. Single Whip (Figure 208-210)

89. Down Posture (Figure 211)

These two forms together form a sequence. Movements 1, 2 and 3 are Single Whip. Movement 4 is Down Posture.

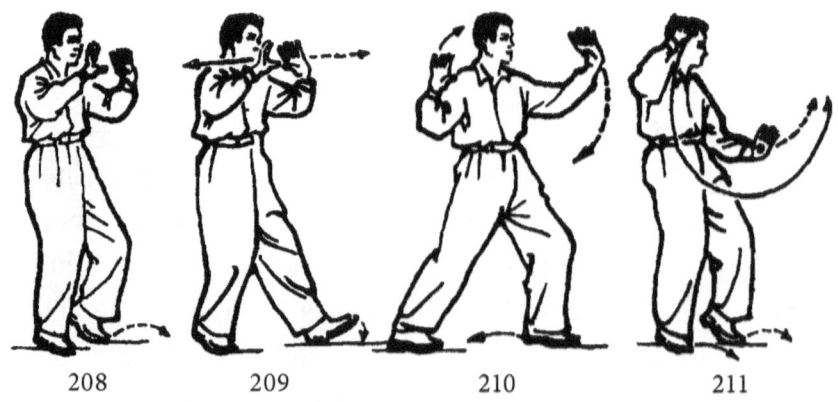

208   209   210   211

Movement 1 and the 56th form turning around Single Whip are the same, and the key points are the same as well. (Figure 208)

Movements 2, 3 and 4:
The 31st form (Single Whip), and the 32nd form (Down Posture) sequence and Movements 2, 3 and 4 are the same, and the key points are the same. (Figures 209-211)

90. Step Up to the Seven Stars (Figure 212)

91. Step Back Over Tiger (Figure 213)

92. Turn, Sweep Lotus Kick
(Figures 214.1, 214.2, 214.3, 214.4)

93. Bend Bow Shoot Tiger (Figures 215.1, 215.2)

94. Double Punch (Figures 216.1, 216.2)

These 5 forms together form a sequence. Movement 1 is Step Up to the Seven Stars, Movement 2 is Step Back Over Tiger, Movement 3 is Turn, Sweep Lotus Kick and Bend Bow Shoot

Tiger, Movement 4 is Bend Bow Shoot Tiger and Movement 5 is Double Punch.

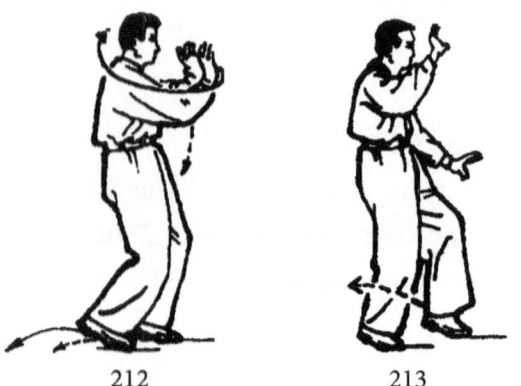

212   213

Movement 1:

(Step Up to the Seven Stars): Look to the east. The left leg steps forward with the heel landing first. The toe points to the east. Next, the body shifts forward and the left leg lands flat with the leg slightly bent. The legs change to left substantial and right insubstantial. Subsequently, the right leg moves up half a step with the toe touching the side of left heel. At the same time, the body turns slightly to the left. When the left leg lands and bends slightly, the left vertical palm extends a little upward. The right vertical palm moves to the right, passing downward by the side of the right hip and then upward to the outside of the left hand. The two hands rise to the front at chest height. The fingertips are at shoulder height. Face east. (Figure 212)

Key points: The movement of the two arms must coordinate with the motions of the two legs. When the right hand is rising, it needs to have the intention of lifting and leading the right foot to step up. After the hands cross, the chest needs to have the intention of expanding. The body must not lean forward or backward.

Movement 2:

(Step Back Over Tiger): Still look to the east. The right leg takes a step back and lands flat with the toe pointing to the southeast. The two legs change to right substantial and left insubstantial. The left foot follows the body, shifting and gathering back with the toe touching the left front side of the right foot. Both arms are also in motion. The right vertical palm rises to the front right side above the forehead. The left hand drops to the front of the side of the left hip with the palm facing down and the fingers pointing forward. Both arms are curved. Face east. (Figure 213)

Key points: After the right leg steps back and lands flat, Spirit must immediately focus on the right leg and accomplish Relax the Abdomen and Tailbone Standing before the other movement can commence. The separation of the two arms to the left and right must coordinate with drawing back the left foot. The body must not rise, and the movement of the two arms should not disturb the principles of Relaxed Chest. Maintain Relaxed Shoulder, and Sink Elbow.

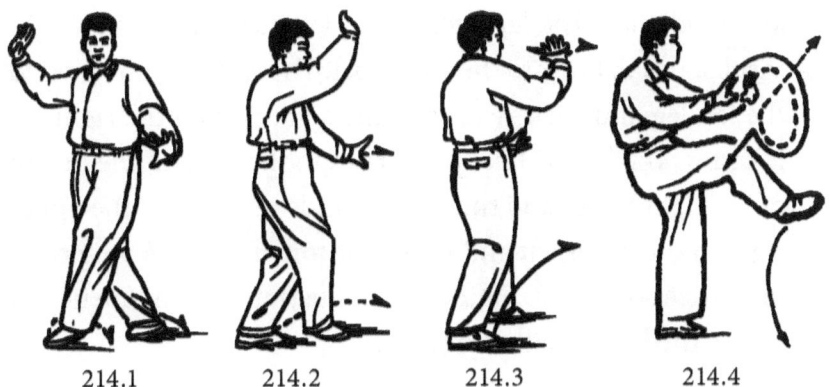

214.1   214.2   214.3   214.4

Movement 3:

(Turn, Sweep Lotus Kick): Lift the left leg and follow as the body turns to the right with the foot landing on the right side of the body to the outside of the right foot. The legs are still right substantial and left insubstantial. Face south. (Figure 214.1)

Following the motion and using the right foot as the axle, the body continues to turn around to the right. The two arms and left leg turn at the same time, when the left toe turns to the east, the right foot lands flat. The two legs are still right substantial and left insubstantial. (Figure 214.2)

Now the left leg takes a step to the northeast with the heel landing first. Next, the right heel pushes and the left leg shifts forward in a curve with the foot landing flat and the body shifting forward. When the right heel pushes, both hands push slowly forward to the northeast. The right vertical palm is at the height of the head and the left palm faces down with the fingers pointing forward at hip level. Face northeast. (Figure 214.3)

Next, the left toe turns to the right, points to the east and lands flat. The legs change to left substantial and right insubstantial. Look to the southeast. The right leg lifts toward the left leg and then sweeps to the right. When the right leg is lifting, the left vertical palm rises to the right at the height of the right hand, and then both hands move from the upper right to the lower left and strike the top of the sweeping right foot. Face southeast. Figure 214.4 illustrates the moment just before the hand strikes the foot.

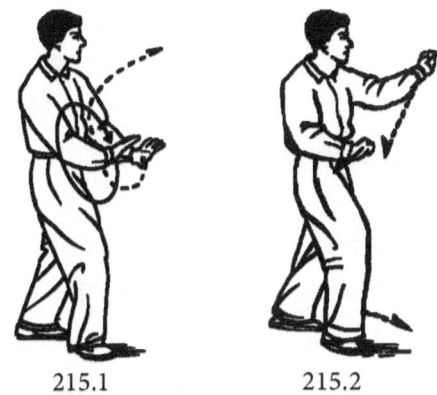

215.1   215.2

Movement 3:

Second half (Bend Bow Shoot Tiger): The right foot lands to the southeast, heel first. Next, the left foot pushes, the right leg shifts forward in a curve with the foot landing flat and the body moves forward. The legs are still left substantial and right insubstantial. When the left heel pushes, both hands drop to the top of the right hip and press down. (Figure 215.1)

Both hands continue to move, gathering inward and slightly downward. Change to the fist in front of the lower abdomen and then lift it to the height of the chest. The body shifts backward with the hands gathering inward. At the same time, the right toe lifts. Look to the northeast. The left heel pushes, the right leg shifts forward in a curve with the foot landing flat, and the body again moves forward. Simultaneously, the left fist, with the palm striking to the northeast, shifts upward to the height of the mouth. The right fist, with the palm facing down presses down in front of the right hip. Both hands are positioned as if pulling a bow, ready to shoot the tiger. Face northeast. (Figure 215.2)

Key points (Turn, Sweep Lotus Kick): Before the left leg starts to lift, both sides of the chest must direct the arms to press slightly forward, following the motion of the left leg lifting. After the left toe touches the ground, it needs to support the right foot to maintain the stability of the body during the turn. When the left leg steps to the northeast it must be supported by Spirit's focus on the right leg. When the right heel pushes, the upper and lower body must move as one. When the left toe turns to the east, the left leg immediately needs to become stable and capable of gathering strength for the right leg to initiate the sweep. During the sweep, the hands can strike the top of the right foot or not, but they need to have the intention of striking the foot. At the same time, the upper and lower body need to coordinate and maintain the Body Principles.

Key Points (Bend Bow Shoot Tiger): When the sweeping right foot starts to land to the southeast, the two upward-moving hands need to connect with the two sides of the chest with the sensation of leading and gathering. When pressing down, the chest needs to relax and sink down to direct the movement of the two arms downward. At the same time attention needs to be paid to the backs of both hands because they need to have the intention of rising. When the body shifts back, it is necessary to have the intention to fold the front and back of the body. When doing the Shooting Tiger movement, both fists must have a sinking sensation and feel the connection between the two arms. The entire Bend Bow Shoot Tiger movement must move smoothly and continuously, with the upper and lower body coordinated.

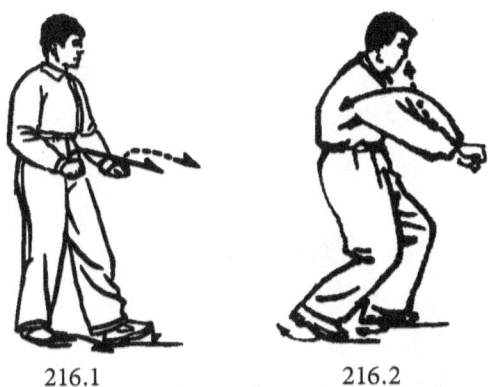

216.1   216.2

Movement 4:

(Double Punch): Look to the east. The legs change to right substantial and left insubstantial. The left leg lifts to take a big step forward with the heel landing first. Both fists drop to the front of their respective hip. Both fists have the palm facing down. (Figure 216.1)

Next, the body shifts forward with the left foot landing flat and the leg slightly curved. The legs change to left substantial and right insubstantial. The right foot moves forward half a step, and the toe touches the side the left heel. Both fists lift slightly upward. As the right foot takes a half a step forward, both fists strike slowly forward and downward, ending with both fists parallel at the height of the abdomen and the arms slightly bent. Face east. (Figure 216.2)

Key points: While stepping, pay attention to the exchanges of the insubstantial and substantial. Jin needs to be transformed internally. The body must not lean to the front or back or to the left or right. When the arms are lifting, they need to have the intention of drawing a curve.

When the fists are striking out, the shoulder needs to relax, and the elbow needs to sink in coordination with the right foot taking a half a step forward.

95. Play the Guitar (Figure 217)

Look to the southeast. Lift the right foot and move it behind the left foot so that it lands flat with the toe facing southwest. The legs immediately change to right substantial and left insubstantial. Next, gather the left foot back with the toe landing next to the left front of the right foot. At the same time, the body turns slightly to the right, the two fists lift and draw a circle with the left and right sides of the chest. The left fist moves from lower to upper, and the right fist moves from upper to lower. Next, the two fists turn to vertical palms and gather inward slightly. The left hand is at shoulder height, and the right hand is at chest height, forming Play the Guitar. Face southeast. (Figure 217)

Key Points: When the right foot is stepping back, the tailbone needs to remain centered. The transformation of insubstantial to substantial must be complete before gathering the left foot back. The movement of both arms needs to be round and lively. Other movements and key points are the same as the 8th form (Play the Guitar). Only the direction and angle are different.

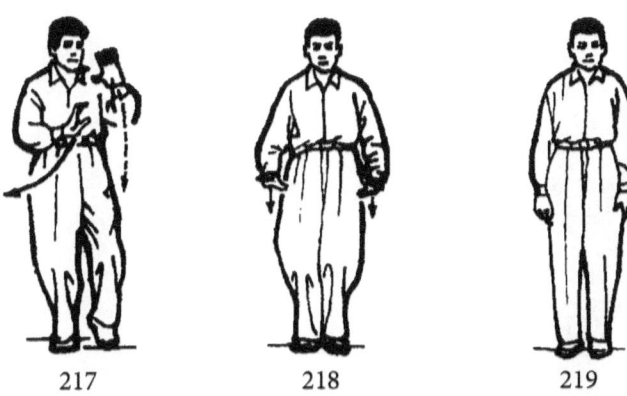

217   218   219

96. End (Figure 218-219)

Look to the east. The left foot comes back and joins the right foot. The body faces forward. Both hands press down to the sides of the hips at the same time. (Figure 218)

Next, both arms naturally hang down like they did at the beginning posture. (Figure 219)

Key points: When the feet are coming together, Spirit needs to focus on the right leg with the left toe still touching the ground. When the two hands are pressing down, both sides of the chest need to relax and sink down. At the same time, the backs of both hands need to have rising intention.

When the body straightens, The Body Principles must still be maintained. When the left heel flattens against the ground, it must be one fist width from the right heel. The toes point slightly out.

Once still, all is still.

CHAPTER FIVE
WU STYLE TAI JI QUAN STRIKING HANDS PRACTICE

STRIKING HANDS IS ALSO called Pushing Hands. However, the term Striking Hands was used by the founders of Wu Style Tai Ji. This book uses the term Striking Hands instead of Pushing Hands because the art of Tai Ji Quan does not rely solely on the use of the two hands to push. There are many ways that the practitioner of Tai Ji Quan can unbalance opponents and make them fall. Thus, the word "push" does not convey or reflect the totality of its capabilities. In comparison, Striking Hands has a more comprehensive and, at the same time, precise, meaning.

STRIKING HANDS
BASIC PRACTICE METHODS

In Wu Style Tai Ji Quan Striking Hands, there are two basic practice methods: Moving Step and Fixed Step Striking Hands.

Wu YuXiang and Li YiYu only passed down the moving step method. The footwork pattern is forward three and a half steps and retreat three and a half steps. On the first and second forward step, the foot should be placed to the outside of the opponent's front foot. On the third forward step, the foot should be placed in between the opponent's feet, and on the fourth step, the back foot should move right next to the front foot with the toe touching the ground. This step is a half-step. Each forward step, whether stepping to the outside or in between the opponent's feet should always land close to the opponent's front foot. When moving in a straight line, either going forward or backwards, the hands and upper body engage in ward off, roll back, press and push. The hands of both participants are in continuous motion during moving step Striking Hands practice.

The reason for using moving step rather than Fixed Step Striking Hands is that Moving Step is more flexible and lively, and therefore presents less reason for concern about stagnation and sluggishness. The moving step footwork and the requirement that one remain centered and balanced while in motion makes it possible to develop the basic skills of Striking Hands: stick, connect, adhere and follow, not retreating and not opposing. These skills teach one how to control an opponent and look for opportunities to express Jin. They also lead to an understanding of the concepts of substantial and insubstantial as well as demonstrating how Jin can be transformed internally. As one becomes skillful, one can embody the ancient motto: "Walking, standing, sitting or lying down, one is always practicing Tai Ji Quan."

When beginning the practice of Moving Step Striking Hands, one must take into consideration the hand movements, the footwork and the requirements of the Body Principles. Often one is only able to control the upper and not the lower body, or is able to control the lower but not the upper body.

Not being able to be in control of both makes it difficult to practice and learn. To make it easier for the practitioner to study Striking Hands in a more gradual manner, I started by teaching Fixed Step Striking Hands. Fixed Step Striking Hands still uses ward off, roll back, press and push with the four hands, but without the moving steps. Once one becomes skillful with the four hands, one can start moving onward to Moving Step Striking Hands practice.

In both Moving Step and Fixed Step Striking Hands, at the beginning, the practitioner must be diligent in practicing ward off, roll back, press and push. Using four hands is also the fundamental method for practicing stick, connect, adhere and follow, not retreating and not opposing. Ask yourself where the opponent touches you and bring attention to that spot. The body must be centered and erect, not leaning in any direction. Jing, Qi and Spirit must focus on the arm. In practicing moving step, one must be proficient in "up and down follow each other." With time and continual practice, one can achieve the fundamental skills of stick, connect, adhere and follow, not retreating and not opposing. From this point, one can find the right opportunity and timing by letting go of self to follow others. "From knowing oneself, one knows others." The skill of "leading to emptiness, borrow force to strike back" will soon be attainable.

This is similar to descriptions from Wang ZongYue's *Striking Hands Sonnet*.

Ward off, roll back, press and push need to be studied in earnest.

When up and down follow each other, no one can enter.

No matter how strong the force,

Steering four ounces redirects one thousand pounds.

Leading to emptiness, unite and the opponent is out.

Stick, connect, adhere and follow, not retreating and not opposing.

RECIPROCAL, INTERCONNECTED RELATIONSHIP BETWEEN FORM AND STRIKING HANDS

To reach the intriguing level of Tai Ji Quan's "others do not know me, but I know others; others are controlled by me, but I am not controlled by others," the key point is that having achieved self-knowledge, one can know others. Practicing form is learning how to understand oneself. Practicing Striking Hands, is learning how to understand others. Knowing oneself comes first. Only then is it possible to know others. Therefore, to acquire skill in the art of Tai Ji Quan, first start practicing form. Having understood and actualized the principles of Tai Ji Quan movement, one is able to start practicing Striking Hands.

Form practice is learning how to arrange oneself. Striking Hands is learning how to change with the opponent. Success in Striking Hands is built on the foundation of form practice. Perfection of the form practice determines success in acquiring the skill of Striking Hands. Therefore, the practitioner must be diligent in practicing form correctly, first learning to arrange himself, and then learning how to know others. This is Striking Hands. If one underestimates the importance of form practice, one will never be able to acquire the marvelous skill of Tai Ji Quan.

The objective of form practice lies in its application. Therefore, while practicing form, one must think of it as implementing Striking Hands with an opponent. Similarly, Striking Hands is not separate from the principles of form practice and, when Striking Hands, one must treat it as doing form. "When there is no one, act as if someone is there; if someone is there, act as if no one is there. Form practice is Striking Hands. Striking Hands is form practice. The principles are the same." Through form practice, one can apply the theories of Tai Ji Quan to Striking Hands, just as practicing Striking hands can elevate one's skill in form at the same time as it increases one's skill in Striking Hands. This back and forth helps to advance one's skill in Tai Ji Quan. Acquiring the art of Tai Ji Quan is dependent on the complementary and reciprocal nature of the form and Striking Hands practices. One cannot be done without the other.

The practitioner must understand the principles described above, follow the rules and study carefully to succeed. From untrained to skilled, from rough to refined, with each day of practice, one improves. Once skilled, one can become even more skillful. There is no end.

WU STYLE TAI JI QUAN METHOD OF STRIKING HANDS (HAO YUERU)

Tai Ji Quan does not rely on physical form but instead on the formulation of Qi space. It is not external but internal. During everyday practice, one must study and experiment with the ways of spaciousness, relaxation, roundness and liveliness. The Spirit needs to be vibrant. The body needs to feel like a balloon that contains within it the energy of preparing to move as well as a feeling of suspension. Whether high or low, retracting or extending, in front or behind, left or right, the arms are nimble and able to move at will. It does not matter if the legs step forward or backward or turn left or right, they are able to transform between insubstantial and substantial, and can move according to one's desire. As one's skill increases, eventually one will be able to reach the realm wherein one is not sure why the hands move and the legs dance. When one understands the principles, becomes skillful with the body methods, knows how to use intention, and is ingenious in moving Qi, every move will conform to the Body Principles. At this point, there is no such thing as wrong.

When learning Tai Ji Quan, one must first seek to center the tailbone. Centering means aligning the end of the tailbone with the center of the face. When stepping to the left, the left hip pulls up slightly, using the right hip to lift it up. Stepping to the right, the right hip pulls up slightly, using the left hip to lift it up. This way the tailbone will be naturally centered. Once centered, it is possible to support the eight directions.

When the eight directions are supported, one can turn at will with strength. Next, distinguish the insubstantial and substantial in the footwork. The insubstantial is not empty of force. Internally there is the energy of prepare to move. Substantial is not holding firm. Internally, Spirit is focused on the intention of lifting. It is important, when using the back leg to push forward, that the legs not be rigid. One must be able to distinguish insubstantial from substantial. If one cannot, it is double weighting. Both shoulders need to relax and open and must release any muscular tension. If there is tension, it means one cannot let go of oneself to follow others and cannot lead to emptiness. Sinking the elbow requires that the tip of the elbow have the intention of sinking downward. Pay attention to the arm and upper thigh. Between them there is the energy of prepare to move. Without this energy, one cannot be nimble. If one is not nimble, there is no feeling of roundness and liveliness. One must also have the energy of protecting the stomach. If the energy is not there, there is no strength for the tailbone to stand, and the body will not have a master to coordinate it. Qi also needs to be nourished. There is no harm in cultivating the Qi and letting it sink to the Dan Tian. Jin needs to be gathered. Jin, pliable and able to store energy in a curve, also needs to converge in the spine. The in-breath is uniting and gathering; the out breath is opening and expressing. Thus, the in-breath naturally lifts and is able to seize and uproot a person. The out-breath naturally sinks and projects a person. This is using intention and not brute force to move the Qi. It is the Dao of Tai Ji Quan breathing.

As a skill, Tai Ji Quan is subtle and intriguing. It does not depend on strength and speed. Strength and speed come naturally. They do not require conscious learning. If one wants to learn this skill, it is best to start with relaxing the chest, opening the back, rounding the buttocks, protecting the stomach, suspending the head, suspending the pelvis, relaxing the shoulder, sinking the elbow, and distinguishing the insubstantial and substantial. Once these are learned, seek to gather the Qi. Collect Qi at the spine and drop it to the waist. Open, so Qi can sink down. From here, seek the energy of movement in stillness (the energy of preparing to move). Movement in stillness is Jing, Qi and Spirit (精，氣，神), which means that Jing, Qi and Spirit concentrate in the space in front of the feet, legs and hands.

Focus where one is being touched. Every inch of the body has Jing, Qi and Spirit. Every inch contains Tai Ji. Next cultivate the skill of moving forward, retreating and turning. The focal point of turning is the waist. When one can turn at will, without losing control, then seek the skill of motion and stillness. In stillness there is emptiness. From emptiness, something comes forth. This is what it means to have intention. Intention should not have a preferred direction; it needs to support all eight directions. When practicing a single form, each movement needs to contain four actions: initiate, engage, express and converge. With each action, ask if the eight directions are supported. If the eight directions are not supported, immediately analyze the situation and make corrections.

When practicing two-person strike hands, intention must precede movement, because the opponent's hands cannot match the speed of one's intention. The opponent's strength cannot match collected (gathered) Qi. If the opponent uses force, intercept his strength with intention. Let his force reach the hair and skin, but not oneself. Borrow his strength. Take advantage of his energy. Whichever direction it flows, strike to that direction. Remember not to use force. Do not focus only on Qi. Not retreating and not opposing, following others means I am in control. When the opportunity and timing are right, one can succeed while seeming to effortlessly follow the flow.

Movement is intention. Stepping without disturbing the Body Principles, the hands move without dispersing the Qi space. While performing every move, ask if energy can be transformed in eight directions. If one cannot transform energy in eight directions, it is necessary to evaluate the situation and make changes. In two-person Striking Hands, to initiate action, first organize the body. Intention comes first. Find the opponent's center and go directly to it. When one's intention just touches the opponent's hair and skin, if the action is appropriate, one exhale and he will be out, uprooted. If the opponent uses force, do not allow his force to express itself. Use intention to borrow his strength. Not retreating and not opposing, follow his force to strike him. This is the ingenious skill of borrowing force and using it to strike back. "Four ounces redirect one thousand pounds." This is all accomplished using intention, not brute force, to move Qi. If one can use intention to strike back, over time intention will not need to be used since the Body Principles will always be correct. On reaching this level, everything becomes effortless and instinctive. If it exists it exists; if it is gone, it is gone. Everything follows the heart's intention.

One does not know why the hands are moving and the feet are dancing.

A practitioner of Tai Ji Quan must understand the theory of Tai Ji. If he wants to understand the theory of Tai Ji, he must be fully attentive when practicing and externally at ease, with the Spirit focused. The Qi space is energetic, the belly is internally vibrant. Tai Ji is the body, the body is Tai Ji, like a balloon, moving forward without protruding and retreating without contracting. The left turn is smooth, and the right turn is balanced. It does not matter what the circumstance, there is no discontinuity. All is one. External and internal, form and Spirit, all is forgotten. Enter the realm of subtlety.

In Striking Hands, one's intention needs to come first. Wherever the opponent's force lands, one's intention is utilized there. By the time his force touches one's skin and hair, one's intention has already penetrated to his bone. By using intention and not force to oppose him, and by being neither ahead nor behind, one's intention merges with his force. Left is heavy and then left becomes insubstantial; right is heavy and then right becomes light, rising by going higher, falling by going deeper. Going forward, continue to extend, retreating, continue to recede. Not a feather can be added, nor can a fly land. Others do not know me; I alone know others. This is the meaning of stick, connect, adhere and follow, not retreating and not opposing.

Practitioners of Tai Ji Quan must understand the complementary nature of Yin and Yang. In movement it opens, in stillness it converges. Opening is expansion, growing but not opposing. Converging is contracting, getting smaller, but not avoiding. Between them, Yin and Yang Qi transform, mutually responding, never separating. When one part moves, all move; when one part is still all are still. What is it that moves? It is Qi transforming. What is still? It is the energy of preparing to move. Movement has the appearance of stillness, and stillness has the appearance of moving. Qi is like a wheel, and the waist is like the hub. Hands and body do not move randomly. The key is the Jin gathering. Gather Jin like pulling a bow, express Jin like shooting an arrow. If Jin is not gathered, power is not available to shoot an arrow. When expressing Jin, up and down must follow each other. Jin is initiated from the heel, fills the waist and appears in the fingers. The progression from foot to leg to waist to fingers needs to be one fluid movement. The waist is like the grip of the bow; the hand and foot are like the tips of the bow. Internally it must be pliable and springlike to have the power to release an arrow. When the opponent touches one's skin and hair, one must organize oneself, using intention to receive his Jin. Touching skin and hair means not retreating and not opposing. Using intention to receive is the energy of following. If one can follow, one can borrow force. Once borrowed, the force can be used to strike back. This is: "Borrowing force to strike back, four ounces redirect one thousand pounds." Upon reaching this level, one will unfailingly have the sensitivity to gauge the opponent's Jin and measure its depth. Going forward or retreating, moving to the left or to the right, every move is just right. This is the meaning of: "Know oneself and know others. In one hundred battles, one will win one hundred times." When practicing form and Striking Hands, one needs to understand that form practice is Striking Hands and Striking Hands is form practice. Both use the same principles. In form practice, each form needs to include four actions: initiate, engage, express and converge. In each action one must ask oneself if it is done correctly. If it has not been done correctly, immediately make improvements. "Miss by an inch, miss by a mile." Upon understanding this objective, everyday life (movement, being still, sitting or lying down) becomes Tai Ji. The practitioner must have a clear understanding of this.

When practicing form, one must use intention and not force (i.e. holding the breath or otherwise controlling the breath) to cause the Qi to sink to the Dan Tian. Instead, use gather, nourish and store, without letting the Qi rise. Relax the abdomen with Qi energy vibrant and ready. Practicing this way over time makes it possible to gather Qi to the bone. Afterwards, using intention, pass the Qi from the spine to the tailbone and upward to the Dan Tian. When one reaches this level, one can use intention to move the Qi throughout the body. Wherever the opponent touches, intention focuses there. Qi will flow out from there, like an echo, fast as an electrical shock. Everywhere in the body it is the same, this is the meaning of: "Moving Qi though the nine-hole pearl, one is able to penetrate the slightest void. Move Jin like tempered steel, and nothing can stand in its way. When intention initiates, Qi arrives."

The Qi of the Dan Tian needs to be nourished. This way it is like a long river or a vast ocean. One can use it without diminishing it, take from it without depleting it. Once one becomes skillful, the body will unite as one, like a balloon. If the left is heavy, the left becomes insubstantial; if the right is heavy, the right becomes light. As things appear, flow with them. Everything is just right. Everything arises from using intention and not brute force to move Qi. All is internal, not external. Well-nourished Qi becomes tempered steel.

LEADING TO EMPTINESS, BORROW FORCE TO STRIKE BACK

Tai Ji Quan is an art and not just pure technique, and borrowing strength to strike back is the fundamental uniqueness of the art of Tai Ji Quan.

In Tai Ji Quan, Striking Hands does not depend on one's own strength and speed. Power is borrowed from the opponent by using intention. By borrowing, one uses less effort and one is not harmed. Tai Ji Quan is a style of martial art that emphasizes using minimal physical strength for self-defense. This is what it means to borrow force to strike back.

Borrowing strength is the basic mechanism of Tai Ji Quan kinetics. Our natural-born abilities are limited and will weaken with age. The learned skill can be used repeatedly without depleting it, and thus the art and skill will be long-lasting.

This skill has the intriguing aspect of "four ounces redirect one thousand pounds." If one can use four ounces to redirect one thousand pounds, it means that one can use very little force to overcome greater force coming from others. Thus, an old man can defeat a younger and stronger person. The practitioner of Tai Ji Quan does not need to be concerned about his actual physical strength or age, but instead can focus on the skill of "leading to emptiness, four ounces redirect one thousand pounds."

When the practitioner first reads this saying, he often feels it is very deep and incomprehensible and does not know how to begin to acquire this skill. In fact, by following the principles and studying consistently, upon reaching a certain level of skill, it will gradually become clear. Eventually it will become reality. From familiarity comes a gradual understanding. Understanding eventually becomes intuitive and natural.

The practitioner of Tai Ji must remember the principle of using intention and not force. The intriguing part of Striking Hands lies in using intention. Each movement is not just a simple physical motion. First there is initiation of intention, then Qi moves, and the physical form begins. Although one needs to clearly separate intention and Qi, they also work together. Intention is the leader and moves the Qi. When intention arises, Qi arrives. With intention and Qi working together seamlessly, one can discover the captivating aspect of leading to emptiness. Initiate from the heart (feelings) and then the body. Once Qi is embodied, one can lead to emptiness and borrow force to strike back.

What does leading to emptiness mean? Leading to emptiness means having the courage to let the opponent in, not trying to stop him from entering. Only when one has the courage to let the opponent in is leading to emptiness possible. Without letting the opponent in, it is not possible to lead to emptiness.

Letting the opponent in has a premise: Although one is letting the opponent in, one is using one's intention to steer him inward. This requires stick, connect, adhere and follow, not retreating, not forcing. With the right opportunity and timing, one lets go of oneself and follows the opponent, understanding oneself and the opponent. Even if the opponent is fast, he cannot get ahead of one's intention. Even if the opponent is stronger, he is not as strong as collected Qi. If the opponent strikes fast and forcefully, one's intention has already received it ahead of time. Follow him, seize his Jin, not ahead or behind. Borrow his force completely by leading it and simultaneously gathering it. Once gathered, then project. "Leading to emptiness. Borrowing force to strike back" will then be possible. Do not use physical force exclusively, and do not depend only on Qi. Intention and Qi need to work together seamlessly.

Wherever the opponent touches, Intention is placed there. One needs to know oneself and the opponent. If one wants to know the opponent, one must remain unknown to the opponent and use one's insubstantiality to explore the substantiality of the opponent's Jin. One must gauge the magnitude, depth and thickness of his Jin. If the left is heavy, the left becomes insubstantial, if the right is heavy, the right becomes light. Avoid the opponent's substantial and enter his insubstantial. Follow his energy, borrow his force. This is what it means to know oneself and know others. "One will win one hundred battles one hundred times." Only by knowing oneself and knowing others is it possible to move and shift with the opponent. Once able to move and shift with the opponent, the skill of leading to emptiness, "four ounces redirect one thousand pounds" becomes something fascinating to behold.

If one wants to know oneself and know others, one must first start with letting go of oneself and following others, not imposing oneself on others. Following others is lively, following oneself is stagnation. However, one must follow the other in such a way as to gain control over the other.

If the opponent wants to go to the left, use intention to lead him to the left; if the opponent wants to go to the right, use intention to lead him to the right; if he wants to advance forward, use intention to steer him forward; if he wants to retreat, use intention to follow him; if he wants to go up, use intention to assist him upwards; if he wants to go down, use intention to assist him downward; if he wants to open, use intention to help him open; if he wants to close, use intention to help him close. When reaching this level, one can actualize "if left is heavy, left becomes insubstantial; if right is heavy, right becomes light; rise by going higher; descend by going deeper; going forward, continue to extend; retreating, continue to recede." Seen from the outside, it appears that one is following the opponent, however, the opponent is controlled by one's own internal energy. Therefore, letting go of oneself to follow others is actually being in control. Letting oneself follow others is not externally following their movements. If there is no internal form to direct the action, it is letting go of what is immediate and searching for something far away. By doing so, one cannot satisfy the requirement of letting go of oneself and following others. Instead, the opponent can find an opening to enter. Thus, letting go of oneself and following others must combine both the internal and external. The key point is internal. Only when one can let go of oneself and follow others can one discover the insubstantiality or substantiality of the opponents Jin.

The body's Jin lies in its unification. The body's Qi lies in its convergence (gathering). Each of the Body Principles must be applied and unified before pursuing the convergence of the Qi. Qi needs to converge (gather) at the lower back. Convergence means that one must use intention to let Qi sink and stick to the back. From both shoulders, gather Qi to the spine so that it converges at the lower back. Once Qi converges at the lower back, then let it fill the waist. Qi space needs to surround Spirit; Spirit needs to support Qi space. With Spirit gathered, Qi converged and the mind focused, Jing, Qi, and Spirit, become one. If one moves, all move. If one is still, all are still. One must organize oneself when the opponent engages. From below obtain the opportunity, from above obtain the timing. Up and down follow each other. The power of the front, back, left and right is ready. When the opportunity and timing are right, it is possible to let go of oneself and follow the other.

When practicing Striking Hands, one must make the effort to learn how to stick, connect, adhere and follow, not retreat and not oppose. Moving away is sticking, sticking is moving away. Sticking uses intention, moving away uses Qi. To let oneself follow others, one must know oneself. Only then is it possible to receive and transform. Letting others stick to oneself, one must know the other. Then it is possible not to be behind or ahead. Based on the opponent's strength, one's intention becomes synchronized with it. If the opponent increases, one increases; if the opponent decreases, one decreases, matching precisely. Do not provide any opportunity for the opponent to use strength. He is above and has no place to use his Jin; he is below and has no place to insert his strength. Take the opportunity to enter and receive his Jin. He will fall without fail.

If it is possible to stick to someone, it is possible to seize him, so that he cannot move away. Upon seizing someone, it is possible to use intention to steer him onward to emptiness. If one desires to have something float away, one must push downward to increase the force of rising. The root will be broken, and there will be nowhere to root or stand. As the river and ocean are able to float a ship, the opponent's body can naturally be floated. Once he is floating, he can naturally drift away and be projected. It is done with ease. Remember, borrowing force to strike back must sever his root. If his root is not broken, the force has not been borrowed and cannot be projected. If his root is broken with clarity and sharpness, striking an opponent requires little effort. Without doubt, the opponent will be willing to admit defeat.

If one desires to unbalance someone, one must add the intention of prying up. Combined with leading, transforming and gathering, this naturally can make one's opponent feel like he is falling into an abyss and becoming empty, his Jin received, captured and controlled by another. His center of gravity is lifted up, and his Jin is completely borrowed. With one exhale he is out. As for how far and what way he falls, all can be accomplished by following the energy. This intriguing aspect of borrowing force to strike back comes from "leading to emptiness, four ounces redirect one thousand pounds."

During the practice of every form, ask yourself if there is the feeling of spaciousness, relaxation, roundness and liveliness and whether the Spirit can support the eight directions. If the eight directions are supported, can they be transmuted and transformed? Qi needs to be nourished and gathered so it does not rise. There is no harm in nourishing Qi directly. Qi needs to fill the arms and appear at the fingers. The body needs to be open and full, with all the joints penetrated and connected. Tai Ji is the body, the body is Tai Ji. Everywhere is the same. Move Qi so it can reach all the voids of the nine holes pearl. Qi is like the wheel; the hub is at the waist. Wherever the opponent touches me, Qi arrives there. Insubstantial and substantial are separated there. Insubstantial is Yang, substantial is Yin. Yin does not leave Yang, Yang does not separate from Yin. Yin and Yang are mutually beneficial. In this way insubstantial and substantial can be used to control others.

Remember, the practitioner must use their own insubstantial Jin to explore the opponent's substantial Jin. They must not use their substantial Jin or the opponent will be able to know what is coming. To change and shift with the opponent one must use internal Jin so there is no external trace. Jin is transformed internally so that the opponent cannot gauge it. They can only touch the insubstantial, meaning the skin and hair, and are not able to reach the substantial. Thus, they are not able to use strength. This is the meaning of "others do not know me; I alone know others." Use insubstantiality and substantiality to control the opponent. That way one cannot be defeated. This is attributable to the subtle skill of Tai Ji Quan.

In summary, when leading to emptiness, borrowing force to strike back is using intention to develop a skill, not using physical strength. All parts of the body need to act as one. In movement everything moves. In movement there is stillness, and calmness prevails so that one can practice according to Tai Ji Quan principles. In stillness all becomes still. In stillness there is intention (the energy of preparing to move).

This way, when the Jin stops, intention goes on, so that upon being touched one can immediately project. In openness there is convergence. Upon opening, one can still open more. In convergence, there is opening, so that in convergence one can still converge more. This is "like the long and winding river and the ocean, continuing on, never ending."

It is necessary to clearly distinguish and separate insubstantial and substantial. The transformation of insubstantial and substantial is all internal, not external. When it is internal, Jin can change without leaving a trace. As Jin moves, no one will notice it. This is how one can receive and transform. From obtaining opportunity and timing, to letting go of oneself to follow others; from letting go of oneself to follow others to knowing oneself and knowing others; from knowing oneself and knowing others to leading to emptiness, borrow force to strike back.

To gather Jin like pulling a bow, and to release Jin like releasing an arrow, the body must have five bows. Steer and lead from above; transform at the chest; gather and store at the leg; direct at the waist; gather and then project. Jin needs to be pliable and springlike to gather. Unification is the key to the Jin of the whole body. Projection must focus on one direction, knowing the target, so it can express effectively.

Jin starts at the heel and moves from the feet to the legs, to the waist and the fingers without a break. Every movement must be rounded and balanced, not lopsided. There must be no corners, sharp points or bumps. On reaching this level, it does not matter whether one is moving forward or backward, to the left or to the right. There is no place for others to take advantage. Using intention to move the Qi, using Qi to create Jin, intention rises, Qi sinks. What moves is Qi transforming.

Heart intention comes first and can be applied to the whole body. With time and increased skill, upon inhaling, one is naturally able to lift and thus seize a person. Upon exhaling one naturally sinks and is able to project a person. Inhaling is convergence, gathering and receiving. Exhaling is opening, releasing and projecting. If one practices the principles, in time one will be able to follow the flow with sensitivity. Advancing from here, one reaches the level of "one feather cannot be added. Neither an insect nor a fly can land." There is neither internal nor external. Nothing is incorrect. Every movement follows the principles. Form and Spirit are all forgotten. If the left is heavy, the left becomes insubstantial; if the right is heavy, the right becomes light. On being touched, one will be able to turn at will and conform to one's intent, like an echo, fast as lighting. "Leading to emptiness, borrow force to strike back." Everything follows the heart's desires.

LETTING GO OF SELF, FOLLOW OTHERS (HAO YUERU)

Tai Ji Quan has methods of letting go of self and following others. The place where one is being touched needs to become responsive. If the hand is being touched, the wrist becomes responsive; if the elbow is being touched, the elbow becomes responsive; if the chest is being touched, the chest becomes responsive. Every part of the body is the same.

In addition, if the hand is being touched, the intention is at the elbow; if the elbow is being touched, the intention is at the shoulder; if the shoulder is being touched, the intention is at the chest; if the chest is being touched, the intention is at the waist; if the waist is being touched, the intention is at the thigh. Following this logic, everything such as "stick, connect, adhere and follow, not retreating and not opposing" and "leading to emptiness, borrowing force to strike back" is due to intention.

敷,蓋,對,吞
APPLY, COVER, ALIGN AND SWALLOW: FOUR CHARACTERS SECRET FORMULA EXPLANATION

APPLY: WHAT IS THE MEANING OF APPLY?
Cover oneself with Qi and apply it on top of the opponent's Jin, so he cannot move.

Explanation: Do not use the hand to catch, grab, or seize. Just gently touch and hover on top of the opponent's body. Apply Qi on top of his Jin as lightly as the air, so that the opponent cannot find a place to exert strength. Use Jing, Qi and Spirit to penetrate, so there is no place for him to maneuver and he cannot move.

COVER: WHAT IS THE MEANING OF COVER?
Use Qi to cover where his Jin is coming from.

Explanation: Use Qi to cover his Jin, without alerting him, so that no matter how strong his Jin is, he cannot use it.

ALIGN: WHAT IS THE MEANING OF ALIGN?
Align Qi to where his Jin is coming from.
Target it and go directly to it.

Explanation: This is accurately knowing the direction of his Jin. Use Qi to align to his Jin's location, matching the magnitude, depth and thickness. Employ Jin like tempered steel. Nothing can stand in its way.

SWALLOW: WHAT IS THE MEANING OF SWALLOW?
Use Qi to swallow his Jin whole and transform it.

Explanation: By using one's immense Qi space, surround his body, swallow all his Jin, then transform and dissolve it, so that it does not matter how strong his Jin is, it will all be absorbed.

Additional Explanation: These four characters are ingenious. The body must be as soft as the air, Qi space must become immense. The whole body is like a balloon. There is no weakness. Employ Qi at will throughout the body. Without understanding Jin, it is not possible to reach this marvelous realm. Using the movement of Qi to manifest internal Jin is the meaning of: "Everything is an expression of Qi, no shape or sound."

Additional Explanation Two: Although their usage is different, each of those four characters has its own miraculous effect. Nevertheless, there is an intimate and fluid relationship between them. They are mutually beneficial and can also be exchanged. When all four simultaneously exist in one's mind-intention, they can shift with the opponent. Based on the opportunity presented, they can be flexibly interchanged through the expression of Qi, with neither shape nor sound, thereby demonstrating the marvelous quality of the art of Tai Ji Quan.

WU STYLE TAI JI QUAN
STRIKING HANDS DEMONSTRATION
ILLUSTRATIONS

Since Wu Style Tai Ji Quan's moving and fixed step Striking Hands uses the ward off, rollback, press and push pattern, it is similar to other Tai Ji Quan styles. Therefore, drawings of those patterns are not shown here. Instead, a few Wu Style Tai Ji Striking Hands projection postures are shown for reference.

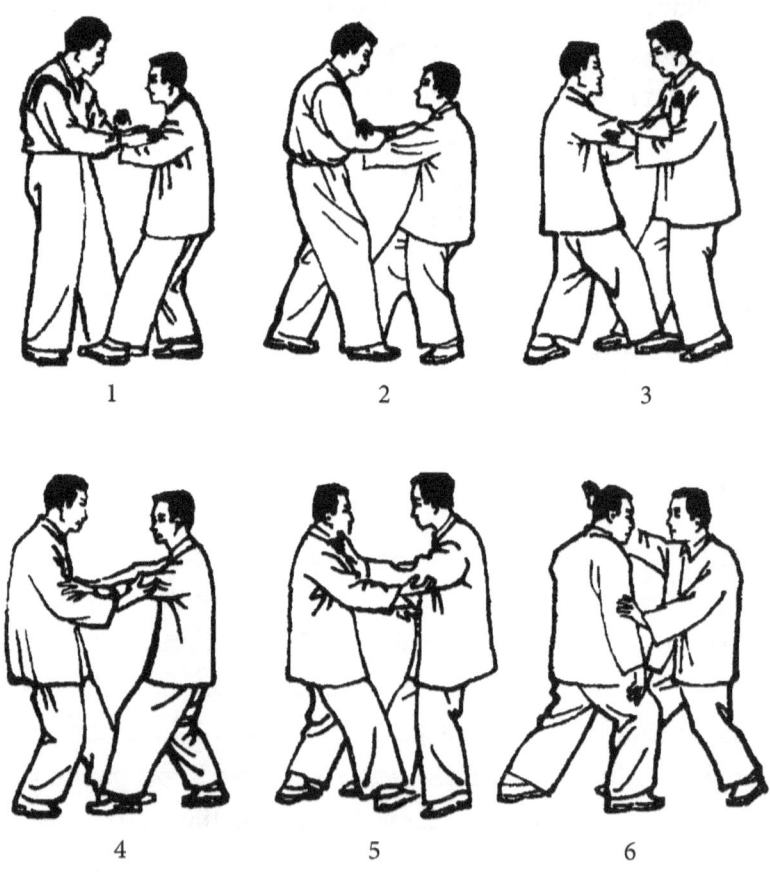

1   2   3

4   5   6

CHAPTER SIX

HAO HE[1]
TREASURED COLLECTION

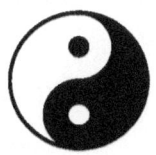

IN 1881
MR. LI YIYU GIFTED
A HANDWRITTEN MANUSCRIPT
OF WANG ZONGYUE'S
"TAI JI QUAN MANUAL"

PLUS WRITINGS BY
WU YUXIANG AND LI YIYU
TO MR. HAO WEIZHEN

---

1 Hao He is the given name and Hao WeiZhen is the self-chosen name.

山右 王宗岳
太極拳論
Mountain Right[2] Wang ZongYue
Tai Ji Quan Treatise

太極者，無極而生，動靜之機，陰陽之母也。

Tai Ji arises from Wu Ji.
It is the essence of stillness and motion,
Mother of Yin and Yang.

動之則分，靜之則合。

Movement separates, stillness unites.

無過不及，隨屈就伸。

Do not overreach, follow the curve to extend.

人剛我柔謂之'走'，我順人背謂之'粘'。

Others are hard. I am flexible.
It is being pliable.
When I am comfortable, others are constricted.
It is called sticking.

---

2 Mountain Right is to the Right of TaiHang Mountain (太行山), a mountain running from north to south, dividing the middle of China. It is worth noting that YongNian County, HeBei Provence where Wu, Li, Yang and Hao lived, is about 100 miles north of Chen Village and the city of ZhaoBao. Both are in Wen County, HeNan Province. The distance from ZhaoBao to Chen Village is about 50 miles and both are about 50 miles from ShaoLin Temple, forming a triangle. In addition, Xing Yi, another internal martial art, was also founded to the right of TaiHang Mountain, about 200 Miles west of ShaoLin Temple in what today is the city of YongJi, ShanXi Province. Right of the mountain is the birthplace of many martial arts.

動急則急應，動緩則緩隨。雖變化萬端，而理唯一貫。

Encountering fast, the response is quick.

Encountering slow, follow in kind.

No matter the change, the principle is the same.

由著熟而漸悟懂勁，由懂勁而階及神明。然非用力之久，
不能豁然貫通焉！

From practice comes familiarity.

From familiarity comes understanding.

From understanding comes knowing.

Knowing comes from practicing diligently over time!

虛領頂勁，氣沉丹田，不偏不倚，忽隱忽現。

Energy rising.[3] Qi sinking to the Dan Tian.

Stay centered, suddenly appearing, suddenly disappearing.

左重則左虛，右重則右杳。仰之則彌高，俯之則愈深。
進之則愈長，退之則愈促。

When left is heavy, left becomes insubstantial.

When right is heavy, right becomes light.

Going up, I am higher.

Going down, I am deeper.

Going forward, I am farther away.

Retreating, I am beyond reach.

一羽不能加，蠅蟲不能落。人不知我，我獨知人。

Not a feather can be added. Not even a fly can land.

No one knows me, but I know others.

---

3 Jin of insubstantial leading upward energy, which allows body to suspend

英雄所向無敵，蓋皆由此而及也！

This is why heroes and heroines are successful
and cannot be defeated!

斯技旁門甚多，雖勢有區別，概不外壯欺弱、快欺慢耳！

There are many practices, although the methods are different.
Mostly it is the strong bullying the weak,
the fast overcoming the slow!

有力打無力，手慢讓手快，是皆先天自然之能，
非關學力而有為也！

Using strength to defeat the weak, slow yielding to fast.
All is based on what is given to us by nature,
It has nothing to do with the study of true power.

察‘四兩撥千斤’之句，顯非力勝；觀耄耋能禦眾之形，
快何能為？

Observe "Four ounces redirect one thousand pounds."
It is not based on strength.
Watch an old man defend himself.
What does speed have to do with it?

立如平準，活似車輪。 偏沉則隨，雙重則滯。

Stand like a balance (scale), lively as a wheel.
Off-center is unbalanced. Double weighting causes stagnation.

每見數年純功，不能運化者，率皆自為人制，雙重之病未悟耳！

After many years of practice, and still not able to transform?
Instead, are controlled by others?
The problem of double weighting has not been resolved.

欲避此病，須知陰陽；粘即是走，走即是粘；

To avoid this problem, understand Yin and Yang.
Sticking is being pliable.
Being pliable is sticking.

陰不離陽，陽不離陰；陰陽相濟，方為懂勁。

Yin does not separate from Yang,
Yang does not leave Yin.
Yin and Yang must mutually support each other.
This is the Jin of Understanding.

懂勁後愈練愈精，默識揣摩，漸至從心所欲。

Once Jin is understood, skill will be gained by practice.
Continue to explore and experiment
until it becomes intuitive and natural.

本是'捨己從人'，多誤'捨近求遠'。 所謂'差之毫釐，謬之千里'，
學者不可不詳辨焉！

This practice is based on letting go of self and following others.
Many make the mistake of not using what is close by,
and they look far away.
The saying goes: "Miss by an inch, miss by a mile."
The practitioner must fully understand those points!

是為論。

This is the Treatise.

十三勢架
Thirteen Principles Form
(Wu YuXiang and Li YiYu)

懶扎衣 Lan Zha Yi, 單鞭 Single Whip, 提手上勢 Lift Hand, 白鵝亮翅 White Swan Spreads Wings, 摟膝拗步 Brush Knee Twist Step, 手揮琵琶 Play Guitar, 摟膝拗步 Brush Knee Twist Step, 手揮琵琶 Play Guitar, 上步搬攬捶 Step Forward Parry, Repulse and Punch, 如封似閉 Withdraw and Push, 抱虎推山 Carry Tiger, Push Mountain, 單鞭 Single Whip, 肘底看捶 Fist Under Elbow, 倒攆猴 Repulse Monkey, 白鵝亮翅 White Swan Spreads Wings, 摟膝拗步 Brush Knee Twist Step, 三甬背 Three Changing Backs, 單鞭 Single Whip, 紜手 Cloud Hands, 高探馬 High Pat on Horse, 左右起脚 Right and Left Kick, 轉身蹬脚 Turn Around Heel Kick, 踐步打捶 Skip and Punch, 翻身二起 Turn Around Jumping Front Kick, 披身 Step Back, 踢一脚 Kick, 蹬一腳 Heel Kick, 上步搬攬捶 Step Forward Parry, Repulse and Punch, 如封似閉 Withdraw and Push, 抱虎推山 Carry Tiger, Push Mountain, 斜單鞭 Diagonal Single Whip, 野馬分鬃 Wild Horse Parts Mane, 單鞭 Single Whip, 玉女穿梭 Fair Lady Weaves Shuttle, 單鞭 Single Whip, 紜手下勢 Cloud Hands, Down Posture, 更雞獨立 Rooster Stands on One Leg, 倒攆猴 Repulse Monkey, 白鵝亮翅 White Swan Spreads Wings, 摟膝拗步 Brush Knee Twist Step, 三甬背 Three Changing Backs, 單鞭 Single Whip, 紜手 Cloud Hands, 高探馬 High Pat on Horse, 轉身十字擺蓮 Turn, Cross Lotus Kick, 上步指襠捶 Step Up, Low Punch, 單鞭 Single Whip, 上步七星 Step Up to the Seven Stars, 下步跨虎 Step Back Over Tiger, 轉脚擺蓮 Turn, Sweep Lotus Kick, 彎弓射虎 Bend Bow Shoot Tiger, 雙抱捶 Double Punch, 手揮琵琶 Play the Guitar.

身法
BODY PRINCIPLES (WU YUXIANG)

涵胸、拔背、裹襠、護肫、提頂、吊襠、騰挪、閃戰。

Relax the Chest, Open the Back, Round the Buttocks, Protecting the Stomach, Suspend the Head, Suspend the Pelvis, Stillness in Motion, Express Jin.

刀法
SABRE METHODS (WU YUXIANG)

裡剪腕。外剪腕。挫腕。撩腕。

Inner Wrist Cut, Outer Wrist Cut, Straight Wrist Cut, Pulling Wrist Cut

槍法
SPEAR METHODS (WU YUXIANG)

平刺心窩。斜刺膀尖。下刺腳面。上刺鎖項。

Straight Thrust to Heart, Slant Thrust to Shoulder, Thrust Down to Feet, Thrust Up to Neck

十三勢, 又名長拳
THIRTEEN PRINCIPLES, ALSO CALLED
CHANG QUAN (WANG ZONGYUE)

長拳者：如長江大海，滔滔不絕也。

Chang Quan (Long Form).
Like the river and the sea, flowing and moving, never ending.

十三勢者：掤、履、擠、按、採、挒、肘、靠，進、退、顧、盼、定，也。

Thirteen Principles: Ward Off, Rollback, Press, Push,
Pluck, Split, Elbow, Lean, Advance, Retreat, Glance Left
and Right, and Center Equilibrium.

掤、履、擠、按，即乾、坤、坎、離、四正方也。

Ward off, Rollback, Press, and Push are Qian, Kun, Kan,
and Li, known as the Four Directions.

採、挒、肘、靠，即巽、震、兌、艮、四斜角也, 此八卦也。

Pluck, Split, Elbow, and Lean are Xun, Zhen, Dui,
and Gen, known as the Four Corners.
Together there are Eight Trigrams.[4]

進步、退步、左顧、右盼、中定，此五行也。

Advance, Retreat, Glance Right, Left
and Center Equilibrium. These are the five elements.

合而言之曰十三勢。

Combined they are called the Thirteen Principles.

---

4 八卦Bagua – the 8 trigrams from Book of Changes denote the 8 directions: North Qian
– Heaven, South Kun – Earth, East Li – Fire, West Kan – Water, NW Gen – Mountain,
NE Zhen – Thunder, SW Xun – Wind, SE Dui – Marsh.

十三勢行功歌訣
Thirteen Principles Practice Sonnet[5]

十三總勢莫輕識，命意源頭在腰隙；
變轉虛實須留意，氣遍身軀不稍滯。

Do not treat the Thirteen Principles lightly.
Intention originates at the waist.
Pay attention to the transformation of
insubstantial and substantial, with Qi flowing
freely through the body without stagnation.

靜中觸動動猶靜，因敵變化是神奇；
勢勢存心揆用意，得來不覺費工夫。

In stillness there is movement.
In movement there is stillness.
Energy shifts magically and changes with the opponent.
Study every posture diligently using mind and heart.
Once acquired, it will seem simple.

刻刻留意在腰間，腹內鬆靜氣騰然；
尾閭中正神貫頂，滿身輕利頂頭懸。

Put the awareness around the waist.
Relax the belly.
Let the Qi come alive.
Center the tailbone.
Spirit rises to the top.
Head suspends the body, becoming light and spacious.

---

5 The original writer is unknown. It could be either Wang ZongYue or Wu YuXiang.

240

仔細留心向推求，屈伸開合聽自由；
入門引路須口授，功夫無息法自休。

Carefully observe how freely
energy contracts, extends, opens and converges.
To enter this door of learning,
personal verbal transmission is required.
From practicing diligently,
understanding will come naturally.

若言體用何為準，意氣君來骨肉臣；
詳推用意終何在，益壽延年不老春。

What standards are used to measure this?
Intention and Qi are the commander,
and bone and muscles are the subjects.
What is the ultimate meaning of this practice?
Longevity and health.

歌兮歌兮百四十，字字真切義無疑；
若不向此推求去，枉費工夫遺歎惜。

This sonnet has only 140 characters.
Every word speaks the truth.
Do not doubt it.
Stay on this path,
or all efforts will be in vain.

打手要言
EXPLANATION OF THE THIRTEEN PRINCIPLES
PRACTICE SONNET
(WU YUXIANG)

解曰：以心行氣，務沉著，乃能收斂入骨，所謂"命意源頭在腰隙"也。意氣須換得靈，乃有圓活之趣，所謂"變轉虛實須留意"也。立身中正安舒，支撐八面；行氣如九曲珠，無微不到，所謂"氣遍身軀不稍癡"也。發勁須沉著鬆靜，專注一方，所謂"靜中觸動動猶靜"也。往復須有摺疊，進退須有轉換，所謂"因敵變化是神奇"也。曲中求直，蓄而後發，所謂"勢勢存心揆用意，刻刻留心在腰間"也。精神提得起，則無遲重之虞，所謂"腹內鬆靜氣騰然"也。虛領頂勁，氣沉丹田，不偏不倚，所謂"尾閭正中神貫頂，滿身輕利頂頭懸"也。以氣運身，務順遂，乃能便利從心，所謂"屈伸開合聽自由"也。心為令，氣為旗，神為主帥，身為驅使，所謂"意氣君來骨肉臣"也。

Explanation 1: Use heart (intention) when deploying the Qi to sink and converge to the bone. This is the meaning of: "Intention originates at the waist." Intention and Qi must be able to change intuitively and efficiently to find the joy in round and lively. This is the meaning of: "Paying attention to the transformation of insubstantial and substantial." The body is centered and comfortable, supporting the eight directions. Move Qi though the nine-hole pearl. Being able to penetrate the slightest void is the meaning of: "Qi flows freely through the body without stagnation."

Projection must be calm, relaxed and focused in one direction. This is the meaning of: "In stillness there is movement, in

242

movement there is stillness." Back and forth require folding; advancing and retreating need transformation. This is the meaning of: "Energy shifts magically and changes with the opponent." Seek the straight in a curve. Gather then project. This is the meaning of: "Studying every posture diligently with mind and heart, put attention at the waist." Lift the Spirit, so there is no worry about heaviness and stagnation. This is the meaning of: "Relax the belly and let the Qi come alive." With energy rising, Qi Sinks to the Dan Tian. Stay centered. This is the meaning of: "Center the tailbone, Spirit rises to the top, head suspends, the body becomes light and spacious." Use Qi to move the body. Be in the flow. All follows the heart's wishes. This is the meaning of: "Energy freely contracts, extends, opens and converges." The heart (intention) gives commands, Qi is the flag, Spirit is the general, the body is the subject. This is the meaning of: "Intention and Qi are the commanders. Bones and muscles are the subjects."

解曰：身雖動，心貴靜，氣須斂，神宜舒。心為令，氣為旗，神為主帥，身為驅使，刻刻留意，方有所得。先在心，後在身。在身則不知手之舞之，足之蹈之。所謂一氣呵成，舍己從人，引進落空，四兩撥千斤也。須知一動無有不動，一靜無有不靜，視動猶靜，視靜猶動，內固精神，外示安逸。須要從人，不要由己；從人則活，由己則滯。尚氣者無力，養氣者純剛。彼不動，己不動；彼微動，己先動。以己依人，務要知己，乃能隨轉隨接；以己粘人，必須知人，乃能不後不先。精神能提得起，則無遲重之虞；粘依能跟得靈，方見落空之妙。往復須分陰陽，進退須有轉合。機由己發，力從人借。發勁須上下相隨，乃一往無敵；立身須中正不偏，能八面支撐。靜如山岳，動若江河。邁步如臨淵，運勁如抽絲，蓄勁如張弓，發勁如放箭。行氣

如九曲珠，無微不到；運勁如百煉鋼，何堅不摧。形如搏兔之
鵠，神如捕鼠之貓。曲中求直，蓄而後發。收即是放，連而不
斷。極柔軟，然後能極堅剛；能粘依，然後能靈活。氣以直養
而無害，勁以曲蓄而有餘。漸至物來順應，是亦知止能得矣。

Explanation 2: As the body moves, the heart needs to be calm. Qi must converge, while Spirit must be centered. The heart (intention) gives the command, Qi is the flag, Spirit is the general, the body is the subject. Careful attention is necessary to acquire this skill. First the heart (intention) then the body. Upon reaching this realm, the body does not know why the hands are moving and the feet are dancing. All flows together. This is the meaning of: "Let go of self and follow others." "Leading to emptiness, four ounces redirect one thousand pounds." One must understand, if one part moves, all move; if one part is still, all are still. There is the appearance of movement, but it is still. There is the appearance of stillness, but it is moving. Spirit is internalized; externally at ease. One must follow others. Do not self-direct. Following others is dynamic; self-direction is stagnation. If one just focuses on Qi, there is no strength. One who nourishes the Qi is pure steel. When others are not moving, I do not move; when others just begin to move, I have already moved. To let oneself follow others, first one must know oneself. Only then is it possible to follow and to receive. To let oneself stick to others, one must know others, then it is possible to not fall behind or get ahead. If Spirit is lifted, there is no worry of double weighting; when stick and follow can be done intuitively and efficiently, it is possible to discover the intriguing aspect of leading to emptiness. Back and forth need to distinguish Yin from Yang. Advancing and retreating need to transmute. Opportunities are obtained, and force is borrowed from others. Up and down must follow each other and coordinate to become invincible. The body needs to be centered and balanced to support all eight directions. Be still like the mountain, move like the river. Walking as though on a cliff, deploy Jin like pulling silk; gather Jin like pulling a bow; express Jin like releasing an arrow. Move Qi through the nine-hole pearl and fill the slightest void. Move Jin like tempered steel, nothing can stand in its way. Shaped like a falcon catching a rabbit, with a spirit like a cat catching a mouse. In a curve, seek the straight, gather then express. Gathering is expressing, engage continuously without a break. By being pliable it is possible to be strong. If one can stick and follow, then one can become agile and nimble. Qi needs to be nourished. Jin needs to be gathered in a curve to flex. Slowly one can respond to all things naturally in the flow knowing when to stop and not overreach to acquire the skill.

又曰：先在心，後在身，腹鬆，氣斂入骨，神舒體靜，刻刻存心。切記一動無有不動，一靜無有不靜。視靜猶動，視動猶靜。動牽往來氣貼背，斂入脊骨，要靜。內固精神，外示安逸。邁步如貓行，運勁如抽絲。全身意在蓄神，不在氣，在氣則滯。有氣者無力，無氣者純剛。氣如車輪，腰如車軸。

Explanation 3: Heart (intention) initiates and the body follows. Pay careful attention to the following: relaxed abdomen, Qi gathered to the bone, Spirit centered, and body quiet. Remember, if one part moves, all move. If one part is still, all are still. They appear still but are moving, and they appear to be moving but are still. Maneuvering back and forth requires that Qi stick to the back and gather to the spine. There needs to be calm. Internalize the Spirit. Externally be at ease. Walk like a cat walks. Deploy Jin like pulling silk. The intention is on gathering the Spirit, not on Qi. A focus on Qi will become stagnant. A focus only on Qi has no strength. Without Qi, it is pure steel.[6] Qi is like the wheel and the waist is like the hub.

又曰：彼不動，己不動；彼微動，己先動。似鬆非鬆，將展未展。勁斷意不斷。

Explanation 4: Others are not moving, and I do not move. If others move a little, I have already moved. I appear relaxed yet I am not relaxed. I appear to be extending yet I am not extended. When Jin is broken, intention continues.

又曰：每一動，惟手先著力，隨即鬆開。猶須貫串，不外起承轉合。始而意動，既而勁動，轉接要一線串成。氣宜鼓蕩，神宜內斂。無使有缺陷處，無使有凹凸處，無使有斷續處。其根在腳，發於腿，主宰於腰，形於手指。由腳而腿而腰，總須完整一氣。向前退後，乃得機得勢，有不得機勢處，身便散亂，必至偏倚，其病必於腰腿求之，上下前後左右皆然。凡此皆是意，

---

6 Wu provided five commentaries on Thirteen Principles Practice Sonnet. The discussions, especially the second explanation, mention that when focusing only on Qi, without a corresponding bodily sensation, there is no strength. With proper integration of Yin and Yang Qi, i.e. nourishing the Qi, the body becomes pliable and strong, like steel. The fourth explanation begins the same way, saying that focusing on Qi alone has no strength. However, it continues by saying: "Without Qi, it is pure steel." There are two potential explanations for this mysterious passage. One explanation is that it is a misprint that happened when converting the handwritten copy to a printed book, and that the word should have been "nourish" to match the second explanation. Or, perhaps it means that once the skill has been learned and has become natural and instinctive, when Jing, Qi and Spirit are integrated and embodied, one can express it without having to evoke a specific feeling of Qi.

不是外面，有上即有下，有前即有後，有左即有右，如意要向上，即寓下意，若物將掀起，而加以挫之之力，斯其根自斷，乃壞之速而無疑。虛實宜分清楚，一處自有一處虛實，處處總此一虛實；周身節節貫串，勿令絲毫間斷。

Explanation 5[7]: In each move, the hand initiates firmly and immediately, becoming open and spacious. It needs to be continuous, not beyond the scope of initiate, engage, transform and converge. If one starts with intention, then Jin arrives. This transference needs to be uninterrupted. Qi needs to be vibrant, with Spirit internalized. Let there be no deficiency, neither lopsided nor intermittent. Rooted at the feet, expressed in the leg, directed by the waist and formed in the finger, from feet to leg to waist, there needs to be no interruption. Advancing or retreating must have opportunity and timing. If the opportunity and the timing are not correct, the body is scattered and off-center. The problem can be found in the waist or the legs or in both. Up, down, front, back, left or right, it is the same. All is intention, nothing is external. If there is an up, there is a down; if there is a front there is a back; if there is a left there is a right; if the intention wants to go up, it requires down intention; if one needs to pry something up, there first needs to be a down force. There is no doubt that the root will quickly sever itself. Insubstantial and substantial need to be clearly distinguished. Every place has its own insubstantiality and substantiality. Insubstantial and substantial exist everywhere. Energy permeates and penetrates all segments of the body. Do not let it be interrupted.

---

7 This is the most famous of Wu's written explanations of the Thirteen Principles Practice Sonnet by Wang ZongYue. The first two stanzas have often been modified and mistakenly attributed to Zhang SanFeng (張三豐), a Daoist who lived in the 13th century. Wang ZongYue was more of a mystical figure who some claim was a student of Zhang SanFeng in the 13th century or who lived in the 15th Century. Some historians even claim that Wang is a pen name of Wu's.

打手歌
Striking Hands Sonnet (Wang ZongYue)

掤捋擠按須認眞,上下相隨人難進。

Ward off, rollback, press and push
need to be studied in earnest.
When up and down follow each other, no one can enter.

任他巨力來打我, 牽動四兩撥千斤。

No matter how strong the force,
Steering four ounces redirects one thousand pounds.

引進落空合卽出, 沾連黏隨不丟頂。

Leading to emptiness, unite, and the opponent is out.
Stick, connect, adhere and follow,
not retreating and not opposing.

打手撒放
Striking Hands Releasing Sound
(Wu YuXiang)

掤上平, 業入聲, 噎上聲, 咳入聲, 呼上聲, 吭, 呵, 哈

Peng-rising flat, Ye-inward sound, Yi-rising sound,
Ke-inward sound, Hu-rising sound, keng, ke, and ha.

太極拳小序
TAI JI QUAN ABBREVIATED HISTORY (LI YIYU)

太極拳不知始自何人，其精微巧妙，王宗岳論詳且盡矣。後傳至河南陳家溝陳姓。神而明者，代不數人。我郡　南關楊君，受而往學焉。專心致志十有餘年，備極精巧。旋里後，市諸同好，母舅武禹襄見而好之，常與比較。彼不肯輕以授人，僅得其大概。

素聞豫省懷慶府趙堡鎮有陳姓名清萍者，精於是技。逾年，母舅因公赴豫省，過而訪焉。研究月餘，而精妙始得，神乎技矣。予自咸豐癸丑，時年二十餘，始從母舅學習此技。口授指示，不遺餘力。奈予質最魯，廿餘年來，僅得皮毛。竊意其中更有精巧，茲僅以所得筆之於後，名曰五字訣，以識不忘所學云。　光緒辛巳中秋念六日，亦畬氏謹識

It is not certain who originated Tai Ji Quan. Its subtleties and ingenuity had been described fully by Wang ZongYue's treatise. Later it was passed on to HeNan state, to the village of the Chen family. In every generation only a few people mastered the skill. In my county, Mr. Yang, who lived at the south city gate loved the practice and went to study it. He was disciplined and focused on learning, and after more than ten years he became skillful. Upon his return, he demonstrated the skill to his acquaintances. My uncle (from my mother's side), Wu YuXiang, saw and liked the practice and often compared skills with him. However, Mr. Yang did not want to teach it and Wu was only able to get generalities.

My uncle heard that in Yu state, HuaiQing county, ZhaoBao City, there was a person named Chen QingPing who had excellent skills. Sometime later my uncle had official business and needed to go to Yu state. On the way he visited Chen QingPing. After studying for over a month, my uncle was able to get the essence and then master the skills. In 1853, when I was in my twenties, I studied with my uncle. He gave me verbal instruction and his full attention. However, I was not clever and after more than twenty years, I was only able to touch the surface. My feeling is there are deeper understandings. To acknowledge and not to forget what I learned, I decided to write down what I have understood and call it the Five Key Words Formula.

Written in 1881, the 6th day in middle autumn, YiYu.

五字訣
Five Key Words Formula (Li YiYu)

一曰心靜: 心不靜則不專，一舉手前後左右全無定向，故要心
靜。起初舉動未能由己，要息心體認，隨人所動，隨屈就伸，
不丟不頂，勿自伸縮。彼有力我亦有力，我力在先；彼無力我
亦無力，我意仍在先。要刻刻留心，挨何處心要用在何處，須
向不丟不頂中討消息。從此做去，一年半載便能施於身。此全
是用意，不是用勁，久之則人為我制，我不為人制矣。

1. Heart – Calm: If the heart is not calm one cannot focus.
Once at the ready, there is no preferred direction, neither
front nor back, neither left nor right. Therefore, the heart
must be calm. In the beginning, each movement is difficult
to control, and it is necessary to study conscientiously. Move
by following others. When restrained, seek to extend (Qi),
not retreating and not forcing. Do not extend or contract on
your own. If others have force, I also have force, and my force
is ahead. If others have no force, I also have no force, but my
intention is still ahead. Pay attention always. Bring attention
to where one has been touched. Seek to understand the ways
of not retreating and not forcing. If one follows this guideline,
within six months to a year it is possible to embody it. It is
about using intention, not using Jin. With prolonged practice,
one can control others and not be controlled by them.

二曰身靈: 身滯則進退不能自如，故要身靈。舉手不可有呆像，
彼之力方礙我皮毛，我之意已入彼骨裡。兩手支撐，一氣貫
穿。左重則左虛，而右已去；右重則右虛，而左已去。氣如車
輪，周身俱要相隨，有不相隨處，身便散亂，便不得力，其病於

252

腰腿求之。先以心使身，從人不從己。後身能從心，由己仍是
從人。由己則滯，從人則活。能從人手上便有分寸。枰彼勁之
大小，分厘不錯；權彼來之長短，毫髮無差。前進後退，處處
恰合，工彌久而技彌精矣。

2. Body – Intuitive (Agile): If one is clumsy, it is difficult to
advance or retreat. Therefore, one must have agility. Use of
the arm must be skillful. When others touch my hair and
skin, my intention is already inside their bone. The two arms
mutually support each other so that they can penetrate at
the same time. If the left is heavy, the left is insubstantial,
and the right has gone forth. If the right is heavy and the
right is insubstantial, the left has gone forth. Qi is like a
wheel. All parts of the body must follow it. If one part does
not follow, the body will be scattered and will not be able to
gather strength. To resolve this problem, seek for the solution
in the waist and legs. First use the heart (intention) to move
the body by following others and not oneself. Afterwards the
body can follow the intention. Directing oneself is following
others. Self-direction without following is stagnation.
Following others is dynamic. If one can follow others, it is
possible to evaluate them and one can unfailingly gauge the
depth and magnitude of their Jin accurately. In advancing or
retreating all is harmonious. The longer one practices, the
more skillful one becomes.

三曰氣斂: 氣勢散漫，便無含蓄，身易散亂，務使氣斂入脊骨。
呼吸通靈，周身罔間。吸為合為蓄，呼為開為發，蓋吸則自然
提得起，亦拏得人起，呼則自然沉得下，亦放得人出。此是以
意運氣，非以力使氣也。

3. Qi – Converged (Gathered): If Qi space is scattered, it is not possible to contain it, and the body is easily dispersed. One must allow Qi to converge to the spine. With no hindrance, Tai Ji breathing becomes instinctive throughout the body. Inhaling is converging and accumulating; exhaling, is opening and expressing. When inhaling, one can naturally seize a person and lift him. When exhaling, one can naturally sink, to release a person. Everything comes from using intention and not strength to deploy and manipulate the Qi.

四曰勁整：　一身之勁，練成一家。分清虛實，發勁要有根源，勁起腳根，主於腰間，形於手指，發於脊背，又要提起全付精神，於彼勁將出未發之際，我勁已接入彼勁，恰好不後不先，如皮燃火，如泉湧出。前進後退，無絲毫散亂，曲中求直，蓄而後發，方能隨手奏效。此謂"借力打人，四兩撥千斤"也。

4. Jin – Unified: With practice, the Jin of the body becomes integrated, and with integration comes the ability to distinguish between insubstantial and substantial. To express Jin, it is necessary to have a source. Jin initiates from the heel, is directed to the waist, forms at the fingers, and expresses from the back with Spirit fully attentive. Just before the opponent initiates his unexpressed Jin, my Jin receives his Jin, not getting ahead or behind, like skin being burned or water spurting out. Advancing or retreating without being scattered, just as a curve seeks to be straight, gather and then express. It will appear easy and casual, but it is effective. This is the meaning of "borrow strength to strike back, four ounces defeat one thousand pounds."

五曰神聚：　上四者俱備，總歸神聚，神聚則一氣鼓鑄，煉氣歸神，氣勢騰挪。精神貫注，開合有致，虛實清楚。左虛則右實，右虛則左實。虛非全然無力，氣勢要有騰挪；實非全然占煞，精神要貴貫注。緊要全在胸中腰間運化，不在外面。力從人借，氣由脊發。胡能氣由脊發？氣向下沉，由兩肩收於脊骨，注於腰間，此氣之由上而下也，謂之合。由腰形於脊骨，布於兩膊，施於手指，此氣之由下而上也，謂之開。合便是收，開即是放。能懂得開合，便知陰陽。到此地位，工用一日，技精一日，漸至從心所欲，罔不如意矣。

5. Spirit – Collected: In the end, when the above four practices are mature, it is about Spirit being collected. Once Spirit is collected, it is possible to do the practices simultaneously, so Qi can follow Spirit. Qi space contains the energy of preparing to move. Intention is focused. Opening and converging are coordinated. Insubstantial and substantial are known. If the left is insubstantial then the right is substantial; if the right is insubstantial then the left is substantial. Insubstantial is not without strength. Qi space has the energy of preparing to move. Substantial is not rigid. Intention needs to be focused. An important point is that the transformation of the chest and waist occurs internally. Strength is borrowed from others. Qi is expressed from the spine. How can Qi be expressed from the spine? Qi sinks down from the shoulders, gathers to the spine and fills the waist. The Qi coming from above and going down is called converging. Qi moving from the waist, appearing in the spine, filling the two upper arms and appearing at the fingers, is Qi rising and is called opening. Converging is gathering; opening is releasing. If one can understand opening and converging, one knows Yin and Yang. When one reaches this stage and practices every day, one's skill will increase until all moves with one's wish and desire.

撤放秘訣
DISCHARGE SECRET FORMULA (LI YIYU)

擎。引。鬆。放。
LIFTING, LEADING, RELAXING RELEASING

擎。擎起彼身借彼力。中有靈字。

Lifting – Lifting the opponent's body to borrow his strength requires agility, sensitivity and intuition.

引。引到身前勁始蓄。中有斂字。

Leading – Leading to the front of the body to start accumulating Jin requires gathering.

鬆。鬆開我勁勿使屈。中有靜字。

Relaxing – Relaxing the Jin so that it is not constricted requires calmness.

放。放時腰脚認端的。中有整字。

Releasing – When releasing, the waist and feet are set and require integration.

走架打手行功要言
FORM AND STRIKING HANDS PRACTICE CLARIFICATIONS (LI YIYU)

昔人云:"能引進落空,能四兩撥千斤;不能引進落空,不能四兩撥千斤。"語甚概括,初學未由領悟,予加數語以解之。俾有志斯技者,得所從入,庶日進有功矣!欲要引進落空、四兩撥千斤,先要知己知彼;欲要知己知彼,先要捨己從人;欲要捨己從人,先要得機得勢;欲要得機得勢,先要周身一家;欲要周身一家,先要周身無有缺陷;欲要周身無有缺陷,先要神氣鼓盪;欲要神氣鼓盪,先要提起精神,神不外散;欲要神不外散,先要神氣收斂入骨;欲要神氣收斂入骨,先要兩股前節有力,兩肩鬆開,氣向下沉,勁起於腳根,變換在腿,含蓄在胸,運動在兩肩,主宰於腰。上於兩膊相系,下於兩胯、兩腿相隨。勁由內換,收便是合,放即是開。靜則俱靜、靜是合,合中寓開;動則俱動、動是開,開中寓合。觸之則旋轉自如,無不得力,才能引進落空,四兩撥千斤。

平日走架,是知己功夫。一動勢,先問自己:周身合上數項不合?少有不合,即速改換。走架所以要慢,不要快。打手,是知人功夫。動靜固是知人,仍是問己。自己要安排得好,人一挨我,我不動彼絲毫,趁勢而入,接定彼勁,彼自跌出。如自己有不得力處,便是雙重未化,要於陰陽開合中求之。所謂"知己知彼,百戰百勝也"!

The saying goes, "if one can lead to emptiness, one can use four ounces to redirect one thousand pounds; if one cannot lead to emptiness, one cannot use four ounces to redirect one thousand pounds." These few words describe it all. At the beginning I was not able to comprehend this and decided to write a few words to explain it so whoever decided to study it would have a path to understanding, thus shortening the time to acquire the skill. If one wants to learn "leading to emptiness, four ounces redirect others," first it is necessary to let go of self and follow others. If one wants to let go of self and follow others, one must first learn opportunity and timing. If one wants to learn the skill of opportunity and timing, first the body needs to be integrated. If one wants to have the body integrated, first the body must not have flaws. If one wants the body without flaws, first the Spirit must be vibrant. If one wants the Spirit to be vibrant, one must first lift the Spirit, without its being scattered externally. If one wants Spirit not to be scattered externally, first the Qi must converge to the bone. If one wants Qi to converge to the bone, first the two upper thighs must have strength and the shoulders must relax and open so that Qi sinks down. Jin starts at the heel and transforms at the legs. Qi is relaxed and collected at the chest. Movement occurs at the shoulders and is directed by the waist. What is above is connected to the two arms; below the two legs are coordinated. Jin is transformed internally. Gathering is converging, and expressing is opening. In stillness all is still. Stillness is convergence. In convergence there is opening. In movement all moves. Movement is opening. In opening there is convergence. Having been touched, one can turn at will with strength. Then one can lead to emptiness. "Four ounces redirect a thousand pounds."

Form practice is developing the skill of knowing the self. With each movement, first ask if the body is properly connected. If there is any disconnection, immediately make changes. This is why form practice must be slow, not fast.

Striking Hands is getting to know others. Both in movement and stillness, it is getting to know others. However, it is still about self-awareness. If one can organize oneself well when being touched by others, one need not move the opponent at all. Follow the force, enter and receive the opponent's Jin. He will definitely fall over. If for some reason one cannot gather strength for the task, it is because one is not able to resolve double weighting. The solution must be sought in Yin and Yang and in express and converge. This is the meaning of: "Know yourself and know others. One hundred battles, win one hundred times."

四字秘訣
Four Characters Secret Formula
(Wu YuXiang)

敷：敷者，運氣於己身，敷布彼勁之上，使不得動也。

Apply: Deploy Qi over self and apply it on top of opponent's Jin so that he cannot move.

蓋：蓋者，以氣蓋彼來處也。

Cover: Use Qi to cover source of opponent's Jin.

對：對者，以氣對彼來處，認定準頭而去也。

Align: Align Qi to source of opponent's Jin. Target it and go directly to it.

吞：吞者，以氣全吞而入於化也。

Swallow: Use Qi to swallow opponent's Jin whole and transform it.

此四字無形無聲，非懂勁後，煉到極精境地者不能知，全是以氣言。能直養其氣而無害，始能施於四體，四體不言而喻矣。

These four characters have no shape or sound. Only after one understands Jin and practices diligently until the skill has been mastered will one know that the description is all about Qi. One needs to nourish Qi directly without harm and then express it in the four limbs, there is no way to describe the sensation.

EPILOGUE

Wu Style Hao Family
Tai Ji Quan History

WU STYLE TAI JI was founded by Wu YuXiang. Although there is a short historical reference to Wu Style Tai Ji in manuscripts written by Li YiYu in which he mentions that he does not know where Tai Ji Quan was created, nevertheless, the Tai Ji Treatise written by Wang ZongYue had described its theory fully.

In each subsequent generation of Tai Ji practitioners only a few were able to master the skills. Chen ChangXing at the Chen Village had the skills and Yang LuChan from GuangPing of YongNian County liked the practice and went to study with Chen for over 10 years to acquire the skills. Wu YuXiang admired Yang's skills. However, upon returning, Yang was not willing to share the knowledge. Later Wu YuXiang learned that Chen QingPin in the city of ZhaoBao was also a master and decided to visit him. After studying for slightly more than a month he was able to understand the skills. Li YiYu, who was over twenty at that time, decided to study with his uncle Wu YuXiang. He practiced more than twenty years to become proficient.

The oral history maintains that after Wu learned the skills, he obtained Wang ZongYue's *Tai Ji Manual*, which had been discovered in a salt store by Wu's brother. Together, Wu and Li sought to combine the theoretical understanding derived from Wang's manual and the skills learned from Chen QingPin to create Wu Style Tai Ji, which is unique and in appearance is different from other styles.

The above is an abbreviated history. The details of the relationship of Wu and Yang are not described by Li YiYu. The story goes that Wu, who came from one of the prominent, wealthy families in town, supported Yang and his family financially during the years that Yang went to study. In addition, Yang sent one of his sons, Yang BanHou, to Wu's school to study Chinese literature. However, Yang BanHou did not have the temperament for literature, and therefore Wu taught his style of Tai Ji to him instead. Many believe the small frame Yang style was created as a result of Yang BanHou's study with Wu.

Originally, the name of the practice was Mian Quan (綿拳), soft martial art. The reason for this name is that, unlike most martial arts, which use hard and fast movements, this practice is relaxed and uses the ability to "stick or adhere" to the opponent. As this practice spread, the name was changed to Tai Ji Quan (太極拳). Some attribute the name change to Wang's treatise using the Chinese cosmological terms Tai Ji and Yin Yang to describe the practice. Another story is that a famous calligrapher, after observing the practice, wrote a couplet that included the word Tai Ji in his praise.

It is worth noting that both Wu and Li were scholars and were the first to provide written descriptions of how to train to develop Tai Ji skills. Much of the technical terminology found in the Thirteen Body Principles and many theories have been borrowed and used by other Tai Ji styles.

Hao WeiZhen was a neighbor of Li and was fond of martial arts. He was Li's best student. His favorite weapon was a halberd weighing fifty pounds. Li had hand copied three Wu Style Tai Ji manuscripts (老三本): a collection of Wang ZongYue's, Wu YuXiang's, and Li's own writings. Li gave one of the copies to Hao WeiZhen for him to carry on the tradition. Hao WeiZhen later decided to go to Beijing to teach Wu Style Tai Ji. When he arrived in Beijing, Hao WeiZhen ate bad food and was very ill. Sun LuTang, who was a famous master of the internal arts of Xing Yi and Ba Gua took him in and cured him. In appreciation, Hao taught Wu Style Tai Ji to Sun. Later Sun started to teach his version of Wu style Tai Ji, which is now known as Sun Style Tai Ji.

Hao WeiZhen had a son named Hao YueRu and a grandson named Hao ShaoRu. Both son and grandson became Tai Ji experts and went south to Shanghai and Nanjing to teach and promote Wu Style Tai Ji, while some of Hao WeiZhen's students continued to teach it in the north. This is the reason one might hear that there are Northern and Southern versions of Wu Style Tai Ji. Over the years, YueRu and ShaoRu continued to expand the art and developed innovative ways of teaching such as the four distinct stages in each sequence of movements: Initiate, Engage, Express, and Converge. In 1963 Hao ShaoRu wrote a book to introduce the Wu Style and included excerpts from Li YiYu's handwritten manuscript. In 1994 after ShaoRu's death, a second book written by him was published that expanded on the 1963 book.

During three generations, the Hao family studied and refined Wu Style Tai Ji. To honor their efforts and contributions, the southern branch of Wu Style Tai Ji is often called Wu Style Hao Family (Wu Hao) Tai Ji Quan

Master Liu JiShun was one of the best students of Hao ShaoRu in Shanghai. When Hao ShaoRu was older, he often designated Master Liu as his representative in public events. Master Liu taught Tai Ji in China after he retired from working as a Tui Na[1] (Chinese bodywork) practitioner in a hospital. Later he traveled to the United States, where he taught Tai Ji publicly in the San Francisco area. He later retired to Southern California. Master Liu has two daughters. Liu Dong married Fan Huirong, and Liu Qin married Jonathan Thomas, and all studied Tai Ji with Master Liu. Under Master Liu, Wu Style Tai Ji has continued to evolve. Some of his contributions are eight "Finding the Flow" exercises and the Sword Form. With assistance from Hao ShaoRu, he also revived the Fast Form, which will be briefly described below.

Master Liu JiShun's Contributions to Wu Hao Tai Ji Quan

Tai Ji, like any art, evolved over time. Each successive generation was able to put their imprint on the style. Wu YuXiang and Li YiYu studied together. With what they had

---

1. Master Hao ShaoRu was surprised at how fast Master Liu was able to learn Tai Ji and by the sensitivity of his hands during Striking Hands practice. Master Liu attributed this to his Tui Na training. When doing body work, it is critical to have a sensitive hand to feel and read what is happening with the patient's body. This training is directly applicable to the listening and Qi penetration skills of Tai Ji Quan. Master Liu requires all his senior students to study his style of Tui Na as part of their Tai Ji training.

learned, and working with the Tai Ji Treatise from Wang ZongYue, they created Wu Style Tai Ji. Their best student, Hao WeiZhen, and his son Hao YueRu and grandson Hao ShaoRu were able to expand on the knowledge and wrote *Wu Style Tai Ji Quan* to pass the knowledge on to future generations. Master Liu himself also has contributed greatly to the learning and understanding of Wu Hao Tai Ji. The following are some of his contributions:

Finding the Flow Exercises (無中生有):
The beginning chapters of *Wu Style Tai Ji Quan* emphasize separating, distinguishing and uniting the Yin and Yang Qi in the philosophical sense. The book also provides Body Principles as the key to learning the system. However, the book did not describe exercises demonstrating how to understand and to use Qi. To help the practitioner learn the ways of the Qi, Master Liu has created eight exercises to supplement the original Finding the Flow exercise, which are similar to Qi Gong.

These eight exercises are:
Qi Sinks Down
Finding the Flow Down the Arms
Finding the Flow Down the Legs
Separation of Left and Right
Heaven and Earth
High and Low
Big Circle
Lan Zha Yi

Wu Hao 49 Demonstration Form: In the early days, a demonstration of the traditional 96 Form took twenty minutes to complete. Many people felt this was too long for a demonstration. Consequently, Hao ShaoRu asked Master Liu to create a shorter form, and the result is the current 49 Form which only takes ten minutes to perform. The names of the forms are as follows:

1.	起勢	Begin
2.	左懶扎衣	Left Lan Zha Yi
3.	右懶扎衣	Right Lan Zha Yi
4.	單鞭	Single Whip
5.	提手上勢	Lift Hand
6.	肘底看捶	Fist Under Elbow
7.	左倒攆猴	Left Repulse Monkey
8.	右倒攆猴	Right Repulse Monkey
9.	手揮琵琶	Play the Guitar
10.	白鵝亮翅	White Swan Spreads Wings
11.	摟膝拗步	Brush Knee Twist Step
12.	手揮琵琶	Play the Guitar
13.	按勢	Press Down
14.	青龍出水	Dragon Rises from the Water
15.	翻身三甬背	Turn, Three Changing Backs
16.	單鞭	Single Whip
17.	下勢	Down Posture
18.	紜手	Cloud Hands (2)
19.	單鞭	Single Whip
20.	提手上勢	Lift Hand
21.	高探馬	High Pat on Horse
22.	左伏虎	Left Taming Tiger

23.	右起腳	Right Kick
24.	右伏虎	Right Taming Tiger
25.	左起腳	Left Kick
26.	轉身單鞭	Turn, Single Whip
27.	踐步裁捶	Skip and Punch
28.	翻身二起	Turn, Double Rise
29.	右蹬腳	Right Heel Kick
30.	上步搬攬捶	Step Forward, Parry, Repulse and Punch
31.	如封似閉	Withdraw and Push
32.	抱虎推山	Carry Tiger, Push Mountain
33.	野馬分鬃	Wild Horse Parts Mane
34.	上步懶扎衣	Step Up Lan Zha Yi
35.	單鞭	Single Whip
36.	玉女穿梭	Fair Lady Weaves Shuttle
37.	手揮琵琶	Play the Guitar
38.	右懶扎衣	Right Lan Zha Yi
39.	單鞭	Single Whip
40.	下勢	Down Posture
41.	上步七星	Step Up to the Seven Stars
42.	轉身十字擺蓮	Turn, Cross Lotus Kick
43.	上步指襠捶	Step Up, Low Punch
44.	跟步懶扎衣	Step Up Lan Zha Yi
45.	轉身雙擺蓮	Turn, Lotus Kick
46.	彎弓射虎	Bend Bow Shoot Tiger
47.	雙抱捶	Double Punch
48.	手揮琵琶	Play the Guitar
49.	收勢	End

Wu Hao Fast Form: The original Wu Hao Tai Ji form was a Fast Form. Later the Hao family developed a Slow Form for learning the proper energetics. Some believe that the slower form was developed because many people could not handle the rigors of martial arts training. This is not entirely correct for Wu Hao Tai Ji. When performed properly, the Fast Form is not nearly as taxing for the body as the Slow Form. The Slow Form in Wu Hao Tai Ji helps to develop the energy portion of the system, and, when executed correctly, it is a very strenuous workout, especially for the legs. When the Hao family came to Shanghai, they decided to focus on the Slow Form and forego the Fast Form. Master Liu had a chance meeting with a Wu Hao practitioner who studied at another northern school of Wu Hao Tai Ji. This school still practiced the older style Fast Form. Hao ShaoRu agreed to have Master Liu learn the old-style Fast Form from his friend. Together they made corrections to create a new Fast Form that matched the energetics of the Slow Form that was being taught. The sequence and names of the 81 Fast Form are as follows:

1. 起勢　　　　　Begin
2. 左懶扎衣　　　Left Lan Zha Yi
3. 右懶扎衣　　　Right Lan Zha Yi
4. 單鞭　　　　　Single Whip
5. 白鵝亮翅　　　White Swan Spreads Wings
6. 摟膝拗步　　　Brush Knee Twist Step
7. 手揮琵琶　　　Play the Guitar
8. 左上步　　　　Left Step Forward
9. 右上步　　　　Right Step Forward

10.	搬攬捶	Parry, Repulse and Punch
11.	抱虎推山	Carry Tiger, Push Mountain
12.	斜單鞭	Diagonal Single Whip
13.	肘底看捶	Fist Under Elbow
14.	左倒攆猴	Left Repulse Monkey
15.	右倒攆猴	Right Repulse Monkey
16.	左倒攆猴	Left Repulse Monkey
17.	右倒攆猴	Right Repulse Monkey
18.	手揮琵琶	Play the Guitar
19.	白鵝亮翅	White Swan Spreads Wings
20.	摟膝拗步	Brush Knee Twist Step
21.	手揮琵琶	Play the Guitar
22.	按勢	Press Down
23.	青龍出水	Green Dragon Rises Out of Water
24.	三甬背	Turn, Three Changing Backs
25.	單鞭	Single Whip
26.	紜手	Cloud Hands (3)
27.	單鞭	Single Whip
28.	提手上勢	Lift Hand
29.	高探馬	High Pat on Horse
30.	左伏虎	Left Taming Tiger
31.	右起腳	Right Kick
32.	右伏虎	Right Taming Tiger
33.	左起腳	Left Kick
34.	轉身蹬腳	Turn Around Heel Kick
35.	單鞭	Single Whip
36.	踐步打捶	Skip and Punch Down
37.	翻身二起	Turn, Jump Front Kick
38.	披身捶	Step Back Punch
39.	左踢腳	Left Kick

40.	轉身右蹬腳	Turn Around Right Heel Kick
41.	上步搬攬捶	Step Forward Parry, Repulse and Punch
42.	抱虎推山	Carry Tiger, Push Mountain
43.	野馬分鬃	Wild Horse Parts Mane
44.	單鞭	Single Whip
45.	玉女穿梭	Fair Lady Weaves Shuttle
46.	手揮琵琶	Play the Guitar
47.	右懶扎衣	Right Lan Zha Yi
48.	單鞭	Single Whip
49.	紜手	Cloud Hands (3)
50.	單鞭	Single Whip
51.	下勢	Down Posture
52.	更雞獨立	Rooster Stands on One Leg
53.	左倒攆猴	Left Repulse Monkey
54.	右倒攆猴	Right Repulse Monkey
55.	左倒攆猴	Left Repulse Monkey
56.	右倒攆猴	Right Repulse Monkey
57.	手揮琵琶	Play the Guitar
58.	白鵝亮翅	White Swan Spreads Wings
59.	摟膝拗步	Brush Knee Twist Step
60.	手揮琵琶	Play the Guitar
61.	按勢	Press Down
62.	青龍出水	Green Dragon Rises Out of Water
63.	三甬背	Turn, Three Changing Backs
64.	單鞭	Single Whip
65.	紜手	Cloud Hands (3)
66.	單鞭	Single Whip
67.	提手上勢	Lift Hand
68.	高探馬	High Pat on Horse
69.	對心掌	Heart Palm

70. 轉身十字擺蓮　Turn, Cross Lotus Kick
71. 上步指襠捶　　Step Up, Low Punch
72. 跟步懶扎衣　　Step Up Lan Zha Yi
73. 單鞭　　　　　Single Whip
74. 下勢　　　　　Down Posture
75. 上步七星　　　Step Up to the Seven Stars
76. 退步跨虎　　　Step Back Over Tiger
77. 轉身雙擺蓮　　Turn, Lotus Kick
78. 彎弓射虎　　　Bend Bow Shoot Tiger
79. 雙抱捶　　　　Double Punch
80. 手揮琵琶　　　Play the Guitar
81. 收勢　　　　　End

Wu Hao Tai Ji Sword 36 Form: There are multiple forms using weapons associated with Tai Ji Quan. For Wu Hao Tai Ji the weapons passed down from the masters are only the long staff and the saber. Master Liu again got approval from Hao ShaoRu to create the Wu Hao Tai Ji Sword Form. Master Liu had many friends in Shanghai who practiced martial arts. He studied their styles and incorporated moves from these different styles into the Sword Form. Hao ShaoRu also worked with him to develop the proper energetics so that the Sword Form would be consistent with all the Body Principles. Below are the names of the sequences for the Sword Form:

1. 起勢　　　Begin
2. 仙人指路　Sage Points the Way
3. 繃一劍　　Pull Up and Stomp
4. 欲前返顧　Appear Back But Forward
5. 上步直劈　Step Up and Split
6. 懷中抱月　Embrace the Moon
7. 更雞獨立　Rooster Stands on One Leg
8. 大魁星　　Big Dipper
9. 左右橫掃　Sweep Left and Right
10. 中軍劍　　Center Thrust
11. 昭君出塞　Outward Parry, Thrust
12. 攔路虎　　Tiger Ambush
13. 回師揮舞　Step Back and Sweep
14. 白鵝亮翅　White Swan Spreads Wings
15. 哪吒探海　Fairy Explores the Sea
16. 玉女背勢　Thrust Backward
17. 力劈華山　Split Mount Hua
18. 青龍出水　Green Dragon Rises Out of Water

19. 越女背刺　Reflect Thrust
20. 提劍踐步　Lift Sword, Skip Forward
21. 隼鷹撲兔　Eagle After Rabbit
22. 擎天柱　　Heavenly Pole
23. 六封四閉　Appear Closed But Open
24. 展翅蹬腿　Spread Wings and Kick
25. 吳王試劍　King Wu Tests Sword
26. 旋風飄盪　Drift With the Wind
27. 燕子抄水　Swallow Glides Over Water
28. 挑窗式　　Lift Window Open
29. 飛鳥投林　Birds Flock to Wood
30. 雙飛燕　　Twin Flying Swallows
31. 滿天星斗　Stars Fill the Sky
32. 猿猴獻果　Monkey Offering Fruit
33. 白蛇吐信　Snake Thrusts Tongue
34. 提手上勢　Lift Hand
35. 真君奉劍　Master Presenting Sword
36. 收勢　　　End

About the Author

Pang ChaoSun was born in Taiwan and emigrated to the United States at the age of 13. After completing a Master's Degree in Physics, he pursued a career in business. Although he has studied a number of different martial arts over the past fifty years, in 2000 he made the decision to devote his life to the study of Tai Ji Quan. Since 2004 he has studied with Master Liu JiShun, Grand Master of the Wu Style Hao Family lineage of Tai Ji Quan. Pang ChaoSun currently teaches Wu Style Tai Ji Quan in Santa Barbara, California, where he lives with his wife and fellow teacher Gin Yu.

www.ingramcontent.com/pod-product-compliance
Lightning Source LLC
Chambersburg PA
CBHW030410130626
46549CB00004B/1707